THE HIDDEN MAN OF THE HEART
1 PETER 3:4

Archimandrite Zacharias

THE HIDDEN MAN OF THE HEART

(*1 Peter 3:4*)

THE CULTIVATION OF THE HEART IN ORTHODOX CHRISTIAN ANTHROPOLOGY

edited by
Christopher Veniamin

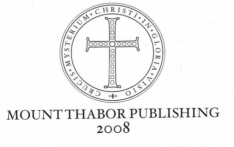

MOUNT THABOR PUBLISHING
2008

First American edition

Mount Thabor Publishing
184 Saint Tikhon's Road
Waymart, PA 18472-4521 USA

www.thaborian.com

Printed in the United States of America

Library of Congress Cataloging-in-Publication Data

Zacharias, Archimandrite.
  The hidden man of the heart (1 Peter 3:4) : the cultivation of the heart
in Orthodox Christian anthropology / Archimandrite Zacharias ; edited
by Christopher Veniamin. -- 1st American ed.
      p. cm.
  ISBN 978-0-9800207-1-7 (pbk. : alk. paper)
  1. Christian life--Orthodox Eastern authors. 2. Heart--Religious
aspects--Christianity. 3. Theological anthropology--Orthodox Eastern
Church. I. Veniamin, Christopher, 1958- II. Title.
BX382.Z33 2008
248.4'819--dc22

                    2007050432

CONTENTS

FOREWORD

Let your adorning be the hidden man of the heart,
in that which is not corruptible, even the ornament of a meek
and quiet spirit, which is in the sight of God of great price

(1 Peter 3:4)

IN THE DEEP OF WINTER 2007 Archimandrite Zacharias journeyed from the Patriarchal Stavropegic Monastery of St. John the Baptist outside the quiet village of Tolleshunt Knights in Essex, England, to the city of Wichita, Kansas in the Heartland of America (Wichita is a mere two hundred miles from the village of Lebanon, Kansas – the geographic center of the continental United States, the actual spot being marked by a tiny Christian chapel). This was the second time (the first being in February 2001) that, at my invitation, Father Zacharias humbly consented to leave his stillness to make a roundtrip of over ten thousand miles to nourish the priests and deacons of my diocese with the rich spiritual fare which is dished out daily at the monastery of his repentance. A spiritual son of the monastery's founder, Blessed Elder Sophrony of Essex (+1993), and thus the spiritual grandson of St. Silouan the Athonite (+1938), Father Zacharias has inherited the rare and precious spiritual gift of 'speaking a word', an authentic word inspired by these contemporary spiritual giants. And what words he brought to us who are children of the late 20th and early 21st centuries!

By God's grace, and the counsels and prayers of his sainted spiritual father, and his own ascetical labours, Father Zacharias has himself adorned the hidden man of his heart with 'that which is not corruptible, even the ornament of a meek and quiet spirit', and his teachings – first made available to the world via audio CDs and now on the pages following – will be easily discerned to be living, fruit-bearing branches firmly attached to the True Vine rather than the dry, withered branches of mere theoretical speculation. The members of our diocesan Saint Raphael Clergy Brotherhood – to which Father Zacharias is so fond of referring as 'that blessed apostolic band' – have unabashedly gorged themselves at the 'rich laden table' laid for us by this godly hieromonk, and have taken great delight in gathering for themselves and their flocks the precious words of life which drop like spiritual pearls from his lips 'at all times and at every hour' in such an unfeigned and even childlike manner. How blessed are you, O reader, to share now in this treasure-trove!

I invoke the blessing of the All-holy and Life-giving Trinity upon this book and upon the 'spiritual meadow' in which it was cultivated and came to fruition (the Patriarchal Stavropegic Monastery of St. John the Baptist), its Hegumen, Archimandrite Kyrill, and those with him in Christ – and most especially one of the two sponsors at my monastic tonsure whom I am blessed to have as a highly esteemed and most beloved brother in Christ, Archimandrite Zacharias.

+BASIL

Bishop of Wichita and the Diocese of Mid-America
Antiochian Orthodox Christian Archdiocese of North America

PREFACE

The Hidden Man of the Heart consists of a series of presentations on the place of the heart in the spiritual life of the Christian, with special reference to the writings of Saint Silouan the Athonite (1866–1938) and Elder Sophrony of Essex (1896–1993). Himself a disciple of the Elder Sophrony, Archimandrite Zacharias bears witness to the golden thread of Tradition passing from one generation to the next, inasmuch as his writings evince that inspiration which is born of the undistorted vision of Christ in glory. As Fr. Zacharias demonstrates with remarkable clarity, it is only in the awakening of the 'deep heart' that the true work of the Christian begins – the cultivation of the human person-hypostasis according to the image of Christ.

About the Author

A member of the Patriarchal Stavropegic Monastery of St. John the Baptist, England, founded by his spiritual father, and translator of Elder Sophrony's writings from Russian into Greek, Archimandrite Zacharias Zacharou holds degrees in Theology from the Institute of St. Sergius in Paris, France, and the University of Thessalonica, Greece, also receiving the degree of Doctor of Theology (Th.D.) from the latter institution for his work on the theology of Elder Sophrony (translated into English under the title, *Christ, Our Way and Our Life: A Presentation of the*

Theology of Archimandrite Sophrony, translated by Sister Magdalen, South Canaan, PA: Saint Tikhon's Seminary Press, 2003). Also, more recently, Father Zacharias authored *The Enlargement of the Heart: "Be ye also enlarged" (2 Corinthians 6:13) in the Theology of Saint Silouan the Athonite and Elder Sophrony of Essex* (South Canaan, PA: Mount Thabor Publishing, 2006).

About the Book

Archimandrite Zacharias' *The Hidden Man of the Heart* constitutes a third book based on his spiritual predecessors, Silouan and Sophrony, and consists of a series of lectures delivered in Wichita, Kansas at the 2007 Clergy Brotherhood Retreat of the Antiochian Orthodox Christian Church. The Retreat was held under the direction of the Right Reverend Basil Essey, Bishop of Wichita and the Diocese of Mid-America on February 6–9, 2007. Each lecture (divided here into chapters) is published in full together with its corresponding *Questions & Answers*.

A Note on Biblical References

For purely practical purposes, the numbering of Old Testament passages has been given according to the Massoretic (Hebrew) text, followed by most English translations of the Bible. The Roman numeral Lxx is used to draw the reader's attention to instances where the Septuagint (Greek) text differs from the Massoretic. New Testament quotations are occasionally corrected in favour of a more literal translation of the original Greek.

C. V.

SAINT TIKHON'S ORTHODOX THEOLOGICAL SEMINARY
FEAST OF THE NATIVITY OF OUR LORD
25 DECEMBER, 2007

INTRODUCTION

THE MYSTERY OF MAN'S HEART

ALL THE ORDINANCES of the undefiled Church are offered to the world for the sole purpose of discovering the 'deep heart' (*cf.* Ps. 64:6), the centre of man's *hypostasis*. According to the Holy Scriptures, God has fashioned every heart in a special way, and each heart is His goal, a place wherein He desires to abide that He may manifest Himself.

Since the kingdom of God is within us (*cf.* Luke 17:21), the heart is the battlefield of our salvation, and all ascetic effort is aimed at cleansing it of all filthiness, and preserving it pure before the Lord. 'Keep thy heart with all diligence; for out of it are the issues of life', exhorts Solomon, the wise king of Israel (Prov. 4:23). These paths of life pass through man's heart, and therefore the unquenchable desire of all who ceaselessly seek the Face of the living God is that their heart, once deadened by sin, may be rekindled by His grace.

The heart is the true 'temple' of man's meeting with the Lord. Man's heart 'seeketh knowledge' (Prov. 15:14), both intellectual and divine, and knows no rest until the Lord of glory comes and abides therein. On His part God, Who is 'a jealous God' (Exod. 34:14), will not settle for a mere portion of the heart. In the Old Testament we hear His voice crying out, 'My son, give Me thy heart' (Prov. 23:26); and in the New Testament He commands: 'Thou shalt love the

Lord thy God with all thy heart, and with all thy soul, and with all thy mind, and with all thy strength' (Matt. 12:30). He is the one Who has fashioned the heart of every man in a unique and unrepeatable way, though no heart can contain Him fully because 'God is greater than our heart' (1 John 3:20). Nevertheless, when man succeeds in turning his whole heart to God, then God Himself begets it by the incorruptible seed of His word, seals it with His wondrous Name, and makes it shine with His perpetual and charismatic presence. He makes it a temple of His Divinity, a temple not made by hands, able to reflect His 'shape' and to hearken unto His 'voice' and 'bear' His Name (cf. John 5:37; Acts 9:15). In a word, man then fulfils the purpose of his life, the reason for his coming into the transient existence of this world.

The great tragedy of our time lies in the fact that we live, speak, think, and even pray to God, outside our heart, outside our Father's house. And truly our Father's house is our heart, the place where 'the spirit of glory and of God' (1 Pet. 4:14) would find repose, that Christ may 'be formed in us' (Gal. 4:19). Indeed, only then can we be made whole, and become hypostases in the image of the true and perfect Hypostasis, the Son and Word of God, Who created us and redeemed us by the precious Blood of His ineffable sacrifice.

Yet, as long as we are held captive by our passions, which distract our mind from our heart and lure it into the ever-changing and vain world of natural and created things, thus depriving us of all spiritual strength, we will not know the new birth from on High that makes us children of God and gods by grace. In fact, in one way or another, we are all 'prodigal sons' of our Father in heaven, because, as the Scriptures testify, 'All have sinned, and come short of the glory of God' (Rom. 3:23). Sin has separated our mind from the life-giving contemplation of God and led it into a 'far country' (Luke 9:15). In this 'far country' we have been deprived of the honour of our Father's embrace and, in feeding swine, we have been made subject to demons. We gave ourselves over to dishonourable passions and the dreadful famine of sin, which then established itself by force, becoming the law of our members. But now we must come out of this godless hell and return to our Father's house, so as to uproot the law of sin that is within us and allow the law of Christ's commandments to dwell in our heart. For the only path leading out of the torments of hell to the everlasting joy of the Kingdom is that of the divine commandments: with our whole being we are to love God and our neighbour with a heart that is free of all sin.

The return journey from this remote and inhospitable land is not an easy one, and there is no hunger more fearful than that of a heart laid waste by sin. Those in whom the heart is full of the consolation of incorruptible grace can endure all external deprivations and afflictions, transforming them into a feast of spiritual joy; but the famine in a hardened heart lacking divine consolation is a comfortless torment. There is no greater misfortune than that of an insensible and petrified heart that is unable to distinguish between the luminous Way of God's Providence and the gloomy confusion of the ways of this world. On the other hand, throughout history there have been men whose hearts were filled with grace. These chosen vessels were enlightened by the spirit of prophecy, and were therefore able to distinguish between Divine Light and the darkness of this world.

No matter how daunting and difficult the struggle of purifying the heart may be, nothing should deter us from this undertaking. We have on our side the ineffable goodness of a God Who has made man's heart His personal concern and goal. In the Book of Job, we read the following astonishing words: 'What is man, that thou shouldest magnify him? And that thou shouldest set thine heart upon him? And that thou shouldest visit him every morning, and try him every moment. . . .Why hast thou set me as a mark against thee, so that I am a burden to myself?' (Job 7:17–18, 20). We sense God, Who is incomprehensible, pursuing man's heart: 'Behold, I stand at the door, and knock: if any man hear my voice, and open the door, I will come in to him, and will sup with him, and he with me' (Rev. 3:20). He knocks at the door of our heart, but He also encourages us to knock at the door of His mercy: 'Knock, and it shall be opened unto you' (Luke 11:9–10). When the two doors that are God's goodness and man's heart open, then the greatest miracle of our existence occurs: man's heart is united with the Spirit of the Lord, God feasting with the sons of men.

We deprive ourselves of the feast of God's consolation not only when we hand ourselves over to the corruption of sin, feeding swine in a far country, but also when we contend in a negligent way. 'Cursed be he that doeth the work of the Lord deceitfully,' warns the Prophet Jeremiah (Jer. 48:10). In the feeding of swine, it is the devil, our enemy, who gives us work which is accursed. But if we do the Lord's work half-heartedly, we put ourselves under a curse, though we may be dwelling in the house of the Lord. For God will not tolerate division in man's heart; He is pleased only when man speaks to Him with all his heart and does His work joyfully: 'God loveth a cheerful giver,' says the Apostle (2 Cor. 9:7). He wants our whole heart to be turned and devoted to Him, and He then fills it with the bounties of His goodness and the gifts of His compassion. He 'sows bountifully' (cf. 2 Cor. 9:6), but He expects the same from us.

From the few thoughts we have mentioned, we now begin to see how precious it is to stand before God with our whole heart as we pour it out before Him. We also begin to understand how vital is the task of discovering the heart, because this allows us to talk to God and our Father from the heart and to be heard by Him, and to give Him the right to perfect the work of our renewal and restoration to the original honour we enjoyed as His sons.

As long as man is under the dominion of sin and death, being given over to the power of evil, he becomes increasingly selfish. In his pride and despair, and being separated from God Who is good, he struggles to survive, but the only thing he gains is a heavier curse upon his head and even greater desolation. But however much he may be corrupted by the famine of sin, the primal gift of his having been created in God's 'image and likeness' remains irrevocable and indelible. Thus, he always carries within him the possibility of a rising out of the kingdom of darkness and into to the kingdom of light and life. This occurs when he 'comes to himself' and in pain of soul confesses, 'I perish with hunger' (Luke 15:17).

When fallen man 'comes to himself' and turns to God, 'it is time for the Lord to work', as we say at the beginning of the Divine Liturgy; in pain, man then enters his own heart, which is the greatest honour reserved by God for wretched man. God knows that He can now seriously converse with him, and is attentive to him, for when man enters his heart he speaks to God with knowledge of his true state, for which he now feels responsible. Indeed, man's whole struggle is waged in order to convince God that he is His child, His very own, and when he has convinced Him, then he will hear in his heart those great words of the Gospel, 'All that I have is thine' (Luke 15:31). And the moment he convinces God that he is His, God makes the waterfalls of His compassion to flow, and God's life becomes his life. This is the good pleasure of God's original design in that it is for this that He created man. God then says to the one who has succeeded in persuading Him that he is His, 'All My life, O man, is thy life.' Then the Lord, Who is God by nature, grants man His own life, and man becomes a god by grace.

In the Gospel of St. Luke we are told that the prodigal son 'came to himself' and said, 'I will arise and go to my father, and will say unto him, Father, I have sinned against heaven and before thee, and am no more worthy to be called thy son' (Luke 15:18–19). This is a wondrous moment, a momentous event in the spiritual world. Suffering, affliction, and the menacing famine of the 'far country' compel man to look within himself. But a single movement of divine grace is enough to convert the energy of his misfortune into great boldness, and he is enabled to see his heart and all the deadness from which he is suffering. Now, with prophetic knowledge, he boldly confesses that 'his days are consumed in vanity' (*cf.* Ps. 78:33). In pain of soul, he discovers that his whole life until then consists of a series of failures and betrayals of God's commandments, and that he has done no good deed upon earth which can withstand the unbearable gaze of the Eternal Judge. He sees his plight and, like the much-afflicted Job, cries out, 'Hades is my house' (*cf.* Job 17:13).

With such a lamentation of despair and, thirsting only for God's blessed eternity, man can then turn his whole being towards the living Lord. He can cry from the depth of his heart to Him Who 'has power of life and death: who leads to the gates of hell, and brings up again' (Wisd. 16:13). This is the turning point in our life, for God the Saviour then begins His work of refashioning man.

When man falls into sin his mind moves in an outward direction and loses itself in created things, but when, conscious of his perdition, he comes to himself seeking salvation, he then moves inward as he searches for the way back to the heart. Finally, when all his being is gathered in the unity of his mind and heart, there is a third kind of movement in which he turns his whole being over to God the Father. Man's spirit must pass through this threefold circular motion in order to reach perfection.

During the first stage, man lives and acts outside his heart and entertains proud thoughts and considers vain things. In fact, he is in a state of delusion. His heart is darkened and void of under-standing. In his fallen condition, he prefers to worship and serve 'the creature more than the Creator' (Rom. 1:25). Because he lives without his heart, he has no discernment and is 'ignorant of [Satan's] devices' (2 Cor. 2:11). As the Old Testament wisely observes: 'The fool hath no heart to get wisdom' (cf. Prov. 17:16), and because his heart is not the basis of his existence, man remains inexperienced and unfruitful, 'beating the air' (cf. 1 Cor. 9:26). He is unable to walk steadily in the way of the Lord and is character-ised by instability and double-mindedness.

In the second stage, man 'comes to himself', and he begins to have humble thoughts that attract grace and make his heart sensitive. Humble thoughts also enlighten his mind; they are born within himself, and they help him in discerning and accepting only those things that strengthen the heart, so that it stays unshakeable in its resolution to be pleasing to God both in life and in death. During the first stage, man surrenders to a vicious circle of destruc-tive thoughts, whilst in the second, inspired by Christ's word, he is led along a chain of thoughts, each deeper than the last: from faith he is led to more perfect faith, from hope to firmer hope, from grace to greater grace and from love of God to an ever greater measure of love. 'We know', as the Apostle Paul says, 'that all things work together for good to them that love God' (Rom. 8:28). Indeed, this entry 'into oneself' and the discovery of the heart are the work of divine grace. And when man heeds God's call and co-operates with the grace that is bestowed on him, this grace summons and strengthens all his being.

When the grace of mindfulness of death becomes active, man not only sees that all his days have been consumed in vanity, that everything until now has been a failure, and that he has betrayed God all his life, but he realises that death threatens to blot out all that his conscience has hitherto embraced, even God. He is now convinced that his spirit has need of eternity and that no created thing, neither angel nor man, can help him. This provokes him to seek freedom from every created thing and every passionate attach-ment. And if he then believes in Christ's word and turns to Him, then it is easy for him to find his heart because he is becoming a free being. His faith is salutary, for he now acknowledges that Christ is the 'rewarder of them that diligently seek him' (Heb. 11:6), that is, he believes that Christ is the eternal and almighty Lord Who has come to save the world and will come again to judge the whole world with justice. He has entrusted himself to 'the law of faith' (Rom. 3:27), and begins to believe in hope against hope (cf. Rom. 4:18), pinning every-thing on the mercy of God the Saviour. Such true faith can be seen in the Canaanite woman, who received the Lord's instruction as a dog receives food from its master, and she followed Him freely and steadfastly. As far as she was concerned, God remained righteous and forever blessed whether He were to rebuke her or praise her. Faith like this receives the approval of adoption because it grows out of love and humility, ever attracting divine grace which opens and quickens the heart.

When man believes and his spirit finds true contact with the Spirit of 'Jesus Christ who was raised from the dead' (2 Tim. 2:8) and Who lives and reigns forever, he is enlightened so that he can see his spiritual poverty and desolation. He also perceives that he is still far from eternal life, and this gives birth to great fear in him because he is now aware that God is absent from his life. Godly fear such as this strengthens man's heart to resist sin and begets a firm resolve to prefer heavenly things to earthly things. His life begins to prove the truth of the words of Scripture: 'The fear of the Lord is the beginning of wisdom' (Prov. 1:7 Lxx). As man's heart draws to itself the grace of God, this gift of fear humbles him, and prevents him from becoming overbold; that he 'not think of himself more highly than he ought to think' (Rom. 12:3), and that he keep himself prudently within the limits of created being.

Another infallible means by which the believer finds his heart is in accepting shame for his sins in the sacrament of confession. Christ saved us by enduring the Cross of shame for our sakes. Similarly, when the believer comes out of the camp of this world (cf. Heb. 13:11–12), he disregards its good opinion and judgment, taking upon himself the shame of his sins, and thereby acquiring a humble heart. The Lord receives his sense of shame for his sins as a sacrifice of thanksgiving, and imparts to him the grace of His great Sacrifice on the Cross. This grace so purifies and renews his heart that he can then stand before God in a manner that is pleasing to Him.

There are many ideas, theories as well as practices, that contribute to the heart's awakening, its building up, its preservation and enlightenment, and finally to its Christ-like enlarging, and we shall develop some of these in the days to come. For the time being, I would just like to mention two more – prayer and repentance.

In the Jesus Prayer, the invocation of the Lord's Name draws the believer into the living presence of the Personal God, Whose energy is imparted to the heart, transforming the whole man. When prayer is humble and accompanied by the practice of watchfulness, the mind is concentrated in the heart that is the dwelling-place of our beloved God, and He grants us a marvellous sense of His closeness that is beyond words.

As for repentance, this all-embracing practice builds and keeps the heart more than any other undertaking. Repentance has a wondrous and holy purpose. The person who repents bears witness to the living God of our Fathers as a God Who is righteous and true in all His desires, all His ways and judgments. But repentance also acknowledges the fact that man is a liar (cf. Rom. 3:4), deluded by sin, and therefore deprived of the honour and glory which God gave him in the beginning. And this is where the person who would repent must begin: he confesses his sinfulness, taking his sin upon himself in humility and self-condemnation. There is no trace of audacity in his conversion, and he becomes true and attracts the Spirit of Truth, Who cleanses him from sin and justifies him (cf. 1 John 1:8–10). As St. Silouan used to say, the Holy Spirit bears witness in his heart to his salvation.[1] But the Lord too is justified, for He is true Who confirms the words of His Prophet: 'The sacrifices of God are a broken spirit: a broken and a contrite heart, O God, thou wilt not despise' (Ps. 51:17). For when man comes to himself and freely says from his heart, 'Father, I have sinned against heaven, and before thee, and am no more worthy to be called thy son', the voice of heavenly goodness then sounds in his soul: 'All that I have is thine' (Luke 15:18–19, 31).

To begin with, man repents of his sins. But as the grace of repentance increases, his estrangement from eternal life is healed and the wisdom of God's pre-eternal design with regard to man opens up before him. The image (cf. John 5:37) of his Archetype, Christ, is gradually formed in his heart as he perceives ever more clearly his calling to become like Him, 'after the image of him that created him' (Col. 3:10) and he no longer compares himself with mortals, but with the eternal God. This vision leads him to the fullness of repentance, that is, repentance on the ontological level, which, according to Fr. Sophrony, has no end upon earth.

In the early stages of repentance, the believer carries the small cross that God's Providence, in His discernment and love for mankind, has foreseen in the life of each one of us. Our personal cross is shaped according to our specific need to be liberated from every form of passionate attachment, and unless we carry it we will never be able to love God our Creator and Benefactor with a free heart and run His course faithfully and steadily. In other words, we take up our cross in response to the commandment to repent, and it becomes the key to our entry into the great and eternal inheritance, which Christ gained for us through His Cross and Resurrection.

But there are no limits to man's repentance. The highest form of repentance for which God bestows an exceptional measure of grace is when man who offers up a cry of repentance for the whole human race and, like another Adam, perceives the cosmic consequences of his own fallen state. We see examples of this kind of repentance in the three Holy Children in Babylon, in the great Apostle Paul, in the humble intercession of all the saints, and last but not least, in St. Silouan's prayer for the whole world: 'I pray Thee O merciful Lord for all the peoples of the earth, that they may come to know Thee by Thy Holy Spirit.'[2] The depth of this deceptively simple prayer can be discerned in *Adam's Lament*, his personal portrait of universal repentance.

How, then, does repentance become universal in its content? If we prepare the soil of our heart with the plough of repentance and continually irrigate it with the living water of grace, a time will come when 'the day will dawn, and the day star will arise in our hearts' (*cf.* 2 Pet. 1:19). At some point, the energy of the Spirit of Truth, which will have accumulated in the heart, will open and enlarge the heart infinitely, and it will embrace heaven and earth, and all that exists. On this day, man will enter into Truth and thus be regenerated as true man. Then, according to the prophetic words of the Psalmist, 'True man goeth forth unto his true work and labour until the evening of his life' (*cf.* Ps. 104:23). He will then know how to 'perfect holiness in the fear of God' (2 Cor. 7:1), to think upon 'whatsoever things are honest, whatsoever things are just, whatsoever things are pure, whatsoever things are lovely, whatsoever things are of good report' (Phil. 4:8), undertaking only such things as will contribute to his spiritual perfecting. The peace of Christ, the Prince of Peace (Isa. 9:6) will reign in his heart, and his every word will echo the treasure of perfection which he contains within himself. He will offer whatsoever overflows from the good treasure of his heart out of love for his fellows, and his enlarged heart (2 Cor. 6:13) will not exclude anyone. His spirit will scale eternal heights and survey the depths of the judgments of God's compassion. He will offer up his prayer, bringing every soul before the Lord, and praying that God may fill the heart of each with the incorruptible consolation of His Spirit.

When the heart is thus given fully to the Lord Jesus, He overshadows it with His messianic power, for He possesses the marvellous key of David, which, with a single right turn, 'brings into captivity every thought to the obedience of Christ' (2 Cor. 10:5). The humility of his thoughts generates intense spiritual energy within him, fuelling the soul's inspiration and endurance in following the good Lord 'whithersoever he goeth' (Rev. 14:4), even to hell. Then again, a single left turn of this key opens the way for all the thoughts of the enemy to return to man's bosom. Should this happen, he will acquire spiritual watchfulness, which will be carried out with angelic precision, making the believer a sharer in the supra-cosmic victory of our God and Saviour. From this point on, his struggle is essentially positive in character, and only rarely negative. The ascetic now labours with ever greater longing 'to be clothed upon with our house which is from heaven . . . that mortality might be swallowed up by life' (2 Cor. 5:2–4), and he witnesses the powerful and infinite 'increase of God' in himself (Col. 2:19).

The heart is now purified by the grace of God, and the mind can establish itself there with ease, through the invocation of the Name of Christ. Whereupon the heart, quite naturally, begins to cry unceasingly with 'groanings which cannot be uttered' (Rom. 8:26). From this time forth, the Lord is ever present, dwelling in our heart, and being 'taught of God' (cf. John 6:45), we learn to discern which thoughts are in harmony with His presence and which ones hinder His coming and abiding in us. In other words, we are initiated into the prophetic life. The heart is instructed to indite good matters (cf. Ps. 45:1), to understand the language of God and with holy determination to cry ceaselessly, 'My heart is ready, O God, my heart is ready: I will sing and give praise' to my Redeemer (Ps. 56:7 Lxx). We are taught how to become signs of the Spirit, witnessing to the truth of Him Who has come to save us and Who will come again to judge the world with justice and goodness. With all our strength, and in all our endeavours, we try to meet the expectations of our Lord, knowing that 'the

Lord loves holy hearts, and all blameless persons are acceptable with him' (Prov. 22:11 Lxx).

I have not said much, but I hope it is clear that man's principal work, which alone gives worth to his life, is the effort of discovering and purifying his 'deep heart', that it may be blessed with the indescribable contemplation of our God, Who is Holy.

QUESTIONS AND ANSWERS

Question 1: Forgive this very naïve question: Where is the heart? Not 'What is the heart?' but 'Where is the heart?'

Answer 1: The heart is within our chest. When we speak of the heart, we speak of our spiritual heart which coincides with the fleshly one; but when man receives illumination and sanctification, then his whole being becomes a heart. The heart is synonymous with the soul, with the spirit; it is a spiritual place where man finds his unity, where his mind is enthroned when it has been healed of the passions. Not only his mind, but his whole body too is concentrated there. St. Gregory Palamas says that the heart is the very body of our body, a place where man's whole being becomes like a knot. When mind and heart unite, man possesses his nature and there is no dispersion and division in him any more. That is the sanctified state of the man who is healed. On the contrary, in our natural and fallen state, we are divided: we think one thing with our mind, we feel another with our senses, we desire yet another with our heart. However, when mind and heart are united by the grace of God, then man has only one thought – the thought of God; he has only one desire – the desire for God; and only one sensation – the noetic sensation of God. That is why repentance and tears are so much appreciated: they help us to find that healing, that state of integrity, because no human being can weep having two thoughts; we weep because of one thought that hurts us. If we are hurt by the thought that we are separated from God, that 'salvation is far from the sinner' (*cf.* Ps. 119:155) and all those things that inspire this pain in our heart, then, of course, we can cry; but if we have two thoughts, we cannot cry. The saints do not have many thoughts; they may have only one thought, but through that thought, they see the whole of cosmic being, heaven and earth. That thought becomes a pair of binoculars through which they see and discern everything. Tears are much appreciated in the spiritual life because, sooner or later, they make the heart surface. If we have tears because we desire God and we want to be reconciled with Him, surely the heart will be found and the mind will descend into it and God will reign there with grace.

Question 2: If a person arrives at that state of having acquired a humble heart, is it possible then to fall back to the old state, and if so, is it harder to get back or is it easier?

Answer 2: We go up and down all the time, but we never stop seeking and 'fishing' for those humble thoughts that unite the mind with the heart. For example, all the thoughts of the Holy Scriptures can help us, because they come from the humble Spirit of God. Therefore, any thought expressed in the Holy Scriptures can become a 'burning coal' that will touch the heart as it touched the lips of Isaiah. That is why we should always study the word of God and have it dwelling richly in our heart, as St. Paul says (*cf.* Col. 3:16). It is easy for grace to ignite one of these thoughts at the time of prayer, and then we have one verse from the Scriptures to pray with for a long time. And the Holy Spirit prays with us because this particular word is given by Him. This single thought that brings tears and repentance may come from the Holy Scriptures, quickened by grace; it may come directly from God Himself, through prayer; it may come from the hymnology of the Church, from a word of an elder or a brother; it can come from anywhere. God is constantly seeking our heart, and He can provoke it with whatever is at hand. We only have to be ready to 'snatch' it. Prayer of self-condemnation is especially helpful. The prayers before Holy Communion are full of these thoughts of self-condemnation before the thrice-Holy God. I think that if we read them carefully, we would always receive great help; one day, one sentence from those prayers will stay with us and work repentance, another day, another one, and so on. Prayer of self-condemnation helps a lot because it follows the path of Christ, which goes downward. He is the One Who first went down, and He then 'ascended up on high, he led captivity captive, and gave gifts unto men' (Eph. 4:8). For this reason Fr. Sophrony says that those who are led by the Holy Spirit never cease to blame themselves before God and this leads them downwards. But we must be careful, because not everybody can bear this. Those who are healthy psychologically can do so and find great strength and consolation, but for those who are less strong, there is another way which involves giving thanks to God continuously, and balancing the prayer by ending it with the words 'although I am unworthy, O Lord'. St. Maximus the Confessor says that true humility is to bear in mind that we have our being 'on loan' from God. We find humility if we thank God continuously for everything, if we thank Him for every single breath He gives us. In one of the prayers before the Sacrament of Baptism, we say that God has spread out the air for us to breathe, and we find a similar idea in one of the prayers of the kneeling service at Pentecost. Consequently, if we thank God for everything and for every single breath of air that He gives us, we will maintain a humble spirit.

Question 3: In our journey to the heart, as we come to know God more, there is spiritual growth. Part of our journey is also learning and studying, and I was wondering if you could comment on the balance between the knowledge and growth of the mind versus the knowledge and growth of the heart. How do we know whether they are growing together or whether they are growing apart? And as we learn, we realize that we will never truly learn anything anyway, and it seems that the heart goes one way and the mind realizes that it will never know it at all.

Answer 3: I think it is true that intellectual work is not very favourable for the activity of the heart, but it is necessary and we have to go through it, at least for a number of years. It is necessary for the life of the Church, especially if we are to serve people. The only thing that can protect us is if we do it in obedience to the Church – to a bishop or a spiritual father. That will protect us and keep us for a time. I remember when I was studying theology, I was trying to keep the prayer. It was not possible. One week I kept the prayer, but the following week I could not keep up with my work. When I tried to catch up with the work, I lost the prayer. I did not have any stability in those years. Sorry, to speak of my personal experience, but looking back, I can say that it was very profitable because I was told to do it and I did it, and the prayers of the one who asked me to do it protected me.

Once I said to one of my elders at the monastery, 'Nowadays, the work of a spiritual father is so difficult and dangerous; you have to be incorruptible to do it.' And he replied, 'No, that is wrong. You do not have to be incorruptible; you have to have a point of reference.' And he was right: a point of reference in the person of an elder in the Church keeps the spirit of humility, that is to say, it protects us from danger. We do not have to be incorruptible, but we have to have a trustworthy point of reference. Nobody is incorruptible.

Question 4: In our modern culture that is so materialistic, scientific and focused on biology and the natural sciences, how can we even become aware that the heart is something more than just a muscle? How can we become aware of ourselves as being something more than just a brain or a circulatory system?

Answer 4: We must learn the language of God. I wanted to talk to you about this later, but I will say a few words now. Because we all have sinned, we all have a common language, the language of pain. When we come to God, we will inevitably have to suffer in order to be purified. If we speak to God with that pain, if we pour out our heart to God with that pain, then God will listen to us, and the heart will be activated. I have an example from the First Book of Samuel. The Prophetess Hannah was childless, but she had a servant who had many children. This servant despised her; she was very proud and arrogant, because she was so vainglorious about her family. Hannah did not take any revenge, although she was the mistress, but she went to the temple and, like one drunk, she poured out her heart to God in pain. Of course God heard her and answered her prayer, and the following year she came back to the temple with her new-born son, Samuel. When we suffer tribulation, pain or illness in our life, we must remember to pour out our heart out to God rather than seek human consolation by going from one person to another and talking about it. This might give us some psychological consolation, but we lose all the tension of life, that energy of pain which is so precious when we direct it towards God. This is one way. The other way, as I have said before, is to find someone who can teach us how to speak to God. In the temple, little Samuel was sixteen or seventeen when he heard a voice calling him and he ran to Eli, the priest of the temple, and the priest said to him, 'Go back to sleep, nobody called you.' The same thing happened a second time. Again he ran to Eli, saying to him, 'Did you call me?' and the priest sent him back to sleep once more. When the same thing happened a third time, Eli, who had been initiated into the life of the Spirit, understood that this was a prophetic calling from God, and he advised him, 'Go, and if you are called again say, "Here am I, speak for Thy servant heareth" (cf. 1 Sam. 3:1-20).' Indeed, the voice called again and Samuel received the prophetic anointing. Similarly, we learn to speak to God with our heart through obedience to our elders and, in fact, the ministry of a priest is to teach his people this language of God in the same way as Eli taught Samuel. We all have a common language of pain, of suffering; one way or another we all go through it in this life, because God loves us.

Question 5: In the monastic life it is easy to see who might be your elders, but how can we identify these persons in our life in the world? From what sources can we find our elders outside of that life?

Answer 5: This has always been an important question in the life of the Church, and I remember St. Symeon the New Theologian saying that one must seek for an elder with tears. Pray to God that He gives you one and, if you do not find one, then speak to God directly, pouring out your heart to Him with tears, and the Lord Himself will be your Teacher. What I say now is a bit risky and dangerous, but it is easy to suppose that there are no such elders any more. I believe that if we are humble, it is easier to find one. If we are humble, we can make anybody a prophet, because if we approach with a humble heart and trust, then God will speak to us. I remember Fr. Sophrony saying to us, 'Make your spiritual father a prophet!' That is to say, approach with faith and trust, and God will inspire him to give you a word. As I have said earlier, true repentance proves that God is just, righteous and blessed in all His ways, and that we are liars. It often happens that we, the spiritual fathers, do not know what we are saying. People come and ask a word of us. Sometimes the word comes naturally without our realising it;

at other times, nothing comes. It does not depend only on us; it depends also on the faith of the person who asks. A little girl, twelve years old, came to me and said, 'Sometimes I have proud thoughts; tell me what to do.' And I said to that little girl, 'Give thanks to God for all the things He has done for you. Give thanks to Him for every breath of air He gives you.' And that little girl grabbed my word and ran away happily. Forgive me for talking about myself, but it is the only way to speak concretely about these things. There is a dangerous side to it, because we can spoil the ethos of our life and of the Church, but I am now speaking among my fellows, among priests, and I feel I can be more specific and open. We must do everything in such a way as not to usurp the spiritual space of the other, of our fellows. And if we are to succeed in this, we have to be careful not to lose our humility.

NOTES

1. Archimandrite Sophrony (Sakharov), *Saint Silouan the Athonite*, trans. Rosemary Edmonds (Tolleshunt Knights, Essex: Patriarchal Stavropegic Monastery of St. John the Baptist, 1991; repr. ed. St. Vladimir's Seminary Press, 1999), p. 304.

2. *Cf. ibid.*, p. 274.

CHAPTER ONE

THE AWAKENING OF THE HEART
THROUGH MINDFULNESS OF DEATH

MAN AND HIS DESTINY were in the Mind of the Triune God 'before the world began' (2 Tim. 1:9; Tit. 1:2; *cf.* Rom. 8:29). At a particular moment which man's limited powers cannot discern, the pre-eternal God decided to create man according to His image and likeness. He made him in a personal and direct way, and endowed him with an incredible mind and a wondrous heart that is capable of embracing not only the whole of creation, both 'seen and unseen', 'visible and invisible', as the Divine Liturgy of St. Basil says, but even the very eternity of God. Man is the true lord of the kingdom of the world, the crown of the whole creation.

From the outset, God endowed man's nature with His own qualities, with every virtue, and with a strong affinity for His Spirit. Man delighted in the good presence of his Creator. His mind could lift itself to God and see His Face, and this vision quickened his heart, which was enlarged with indescribably powerful sensations of unending gratefulness and divine love. Man was so charmed by the greatness of this state that he reached the point of forgetting that he had been created from nothing, and he surrendered to the temptation of disobedience. He wanted to become god, not by means of God's love and in submission to the divine command, but by means of his own independence and rebelliousness. And at that moment, his dreadful fall took place, as the Scriptures relate, and this was a universal misfortune.

Man's mind then cleaved to created things and its vision was obscured. Though its lifting towards God had been lightning-quick, it was now heavy-laden with the sensations of his body. His heart was deprived of the Lord's visitation and all that accompanies this wonderful Presence. He was turned into stone. His mind gradually lost the memory of the supernatural experiences of grace, these being immaterial by nature. Finally, he was bound to the visible world, no longer able to go beyond the immediate reality surrounding him. So did man become unmindful of his Maker, delivering himself up to sin and to its wages of corruption and death.

In this grievous state of forgetfulness of God, man feels an emptiness which cannot be satisfied and a nightmarish insecurity; he tastes of the constriction of death and his soul is oppressed by torment. The passions multiply, filling his being with every kind of vice, and craftily extinguishing all traces of even the memory of God. Man thus becomes incapable of loving, and this inevitably leads him into ever greater estrangement from God and his neighbour, and therefore from the primary purpose of his having been created.

Separated from God Who is the source of Life, man can only withdraw into himself. He is deprived of divine strength and is unable to seek salvation. Gradually he is left desolate and dissolute. Faced by the inexorable threat of his annihilation, man's spirit is seized by the fear of death. He becomes sick with selfishness and enters upon a contentious struggle for personal survival.

When man banishes God and his neighbour from his heart, he loses his sovereignty over God's creation, bestowed on him by virtue of his likeness to God. In other words, he fails in what he has been designed for – to oversee the world with justice and, being enlarged by the spirit of prophecy, to bring all creation to God. He becomes accustomed to living with a deadened spirit, because the hostile power of the wicked one holds his nature fast.

However, God's call is irrevocable and 'steadfast' (*cf.* Rom. 11:29). Furthermore, death is an illegitimate enemy, for the will of God, the basis of man's original issuing forth, has foreordained that man should live eternally 'in immortality' (Wisd. 2:23). Death must therefore be destroyed (*cf.* 1 Cor. 15:26), for which reason the Son of God Himself came into the world to blot it out and to 'destroy the works of the devil' (1 John 3:8). Man's mortality is therefore a phenomenon that runs counter to his nature in that it opposes that for which he has been designed. This is precisely why the human soul is restless: if life leads only to death, then nothing can ever be meaningful.

However, God, Who abides unto the ages and has no pleasure in the death of the sinner, does all He can that 'the wicked [might] turn from his way and live' (Ezek. 33:11). He summons the dissolute from the blindness of their desolation, intensifying by His grace the cruel spectacle of mortality, which entered the whole creation through man's fall into sin. God increases the threat of death by keeping before man's eyes this terrible spectacle. He opens the eyes of the soul that it might behold the mark of corruption and mortality on every created thing. Man then hears the groaning of a universe which has delivered itself up to vanity from which there is no escape. The soul is then granted the grace of perceiving the dark veil of death, corruption, and despair which envelop mankind and all life on earth. This spiritual phenomenon, unknown to modern psychology, is called 'mindfulness of death' in Orthodox ascetic terminology. It has nothing to do with the psychological awareness that we shall die some day; it is more like a deep knowledge, accompanied by a wondrous sensibility of the heart, which perceives clearly 'the futility of any and every acquisition on earth',[1] and that 'all is vanity' (Eccles. 1:2).

This sensibility is produced by the grace of mindfulness of death and in its most acute form all history and world events seem like a mirage, a wicked mockery of man in that true life in God has no part in them, and the dominion of death is everywhere. But when man is enlightened and sees his spiritual state, he also knows that he is bereft of God's living eternity. He is convinced that when he dies, everything that his consciousness has embraced until then – even

God – will cease to be. Man has a deep sense that he was made to live eternally with his Creator, and now he sees that the pre-eternal divine Will remains unfulfilled.

The threat of death, seen as perpetual oblivion, in which the light of consciousness is extinguished, begets horror in the soul and this leads to an unbearable inner suffering. But at this point, man suddenly awakes out of his age-old stupor, for God's eternity summons him from every side. He is as yet unable to face it directly, and there is no suitable place in himself in which to receive it. Nevertheless, his spirit demands eternal life and nothing less can give him rest. He suffers deeply with an intensity that cannot be borne within the limits of human strength. (Many people have this experience before becoming monks and nuns, and that is why they feel the monastic life as an urgency in their spirit. It is not something that they consider carefully and then choose to do; they feel that either they do it, or they die.) But it is then that the most significant marvel in human life can begin: man's spiritual centre, the heart, is revealed.

The disturbing, searing vision of God's absence from creation, now detaches the mind's attention from all created things and earthly ambitions, and calls it back to itself, that is, to the heart. Mindfulness of death is evidently stronger than any passionate attachment, and the mind is now free to descend into the heart and unite with it. This discovery of the heart is the beginning of man's salvation.

When this wonderful grace of the remembrance of death takes up its abode in the deep heart, it draws the mind towards it, and thoughts corresponding to this powerful and awesome experience are born 'from within'. Such thoughts are expressed as follows: 'Everything I know, everything I love, everything that gives me life and inspires me – absolutely everything, even God Himself – will die if I cease to exist.'[2] Similarly: 'In me, with me, all that forms part of my consciousness will die: people close to me, their sufferings and love, the whole historical progress, the universe in general, the sun, the stars, endless space; even the Creator of the world Himself – He, too, will die in me. In short, all life will be engulfed in the darkness of oblivion.'[3] Above all, man is then granted understanding of the futility and vanity of all created things, when they are far from the grace of God. Simultaneously, he is given a deep sense of his inner desolation – the gulf which separates him from God.

Both these disclosures are operations of grace and are extremely beneficial in that they make man aware of his absolute need for salvation. The first, the sense of futility, is accompanied by blessed despair, 'charismatic despair', as Fr. Sophrony used to say, and this liberates the mind from its attachments to the created things in which it tends to wallow. The second disclosure, the sense of his fallen state, inspires his soul with a holy fear of eternal perdition. Eternity then emerges in its negative aspect: man may have met God, but he is still deprived of life in Him. These strange and strong feelings of despair and fear have the salutary effect of humbling his spirit, and bringing the attention of the mind into the heart, the place where God's truth and man's beguilement are revealed. Man can now choose to live according to the will of God. Besides his new and humble fear of God, man also enters into a measure of self-knowledge. If he now embraces the Gospel revelation of Christ as true Being, as He Who Is, as the eternal Victor over death and the Source of Life, he attracts the grace of the Holy Spirit, which unites his mind with his heart, restoring the unity of the faculties of his soul.

This unification of the soul's faculties is the first stage in a man's healing, for he can at last turn to God in prayer, be confident that the sufferings of his spirit will be favourably resolved, and that, in the meantime, God has the power to console him.

But apart from his own tragedy, God 'instructs' man, through mindfulness of death, in the universal aspect of the fall. He begins to see that his sufferings are identical to the sufferings of all humanity. The state of his inner desolation reflects the fallen creation as a whole. He sees, though in a negative way, that he is at the centre of the whole creation which declares nothing but endless vanity. Because he now knows that his being is not limited to his 'self', he begins to love, and this is the prelude to his ultimate regeneration. He now receives strength, by the grace of God, to intercede for the salvation of the whole world, which leads him into authentic spiritual contemplation of heaven and earth declaring the glory of God and the salvation of man.

Mindfulness of death is therefore a gift of God which assists man in finding his heart, which is the beginning of the healing of his person, the purpose of which is to labour for the restoration of true communion within the whole race of Adam. The paradox is this: that mindfulness of death liberates man from the fear of death, and leads him to see all things from the perspective of the love of God. Where death had been a consequence of sin, it is now the Gospel of Life, for it causes eternity to take its rightful place above all earthly things in such an absolute and definite way, that even if the enemy were to offer centuries of earthly bliss and success, the believer now prefers the marks of the Cross through which true joy and eternal salvation are come to the world.

Mindfulness of death unveils divine eternity, but only in its negative aspect. This perception is not, however, psychological but spiritual, and the knowledge it affords is also spiritual, for it simultaneously brings man to twofold vision of the whole truth about himself and his sinfulness. The heart becomes a two-dimensional battleground: on the one hand, man is assured of the existence of the One true God and of His power to save, and on the other, he awakens to a dreadful knowledge of his nothingness, and an indescribable fear of the very possibility of eternal perdition.

Above all, this revelation of eternity, even in its negative aspect, is an encounter between man and the living God. To a certain extent, he draws near to the end of time. Although he feels that his own death, because of his kinship with all of creation, threatens to annihilate all life, at the same time, he accepts the summons to rise up to an infinitely higher form of existence.[4] As he abides in remembrance of death, man perceives in spirit the hell of God's absence. In his desperate desire to resolve this situation, he finds he must detach himself from every passionate involvement with the visible world, and he then single-mindedly casts himself upon God in such fashion as will overcome the passions and, indeed, the very instinct for temporal survival. Self-denial of this kind, inspired by mindfulness of death, creates the best possible environment for ardent prayer to regenerate the entire man, attaching his spirit to the eternal God.

However, an even more astonishing effect of mindfulness of death is a heightened consciousness of the uniqueness of the human person. When man identifies his own personal death with the annihilation of all the life and experience that his conscious- ness has hitherto embraced, as the end of the history of the world, as well as God's relationship with His creation, then the fact that he has been made in the image of God and that his purpose is to be the centre of the whole of God's creation is confirmed beyond doubt. Although the pain of such an experience bears a rather negative character, it nevertheless unites man indissolubly with the fate of his fellows who are one with him by nature, and begets in him a depth of compassion for them, as his salvation now depends on theirs. Such spiritual perception brings man's heart to life, and restores him to communion with the whole race of Adam. When his inner enlightenment attains a certain fullness, and his heart is enlarged and strengthened by divine grace, then the positive experience of love transforms him, for he is now able to embrace all creation and offer it to God in fervent prayer. Then is he led 'into all the truth' (John 16:13) of the love of God, and is made worthy of becoming a true person in the likeness of the New Adam – Christ – in Whose Person 'all things . . . in heaven, and on earth' (Eph. 1:10) are gathered together in one.

Death entered man's life as a curse and grew like a weed because of sin. Christ, however, by His sinless and unjust death transformed the curse into a blessing, and offered man new life in abundance (*cf.* John 10:10). Mindfulness of death introduces man to the greatest wonder this mortal world has ever known. It discloses our own hell, declares and invites us to partake of eternal life. Whoever hearkens and believes, receives that grace which rekindles his heart and brings it back to life. This awakening of the heart is the first step towards the blessed land of everlasting salvation.

NOTES

1. Archimandrite Sophrony (Sakharov), *We Shall See Him As He Is*, trans. Rosemary Edmonds (Tolleshunt Knights, Essex: Patriarchal Stavropegic Monastery of St. John the Baptist, 1988; repr. ed. St. Herman of Alaska Brotherhood, 2006), p. 106.

2. *Idem, On Prayer*, trans. Rosemary Edmonds (Tolleshunt Knights, Essex: Patriarchal Stavropegic Monastery of St. John the Baptist, 1996; repr. ed. St. Vladimir's Seminary Press, 1998), p. 41.

3. *Op. cit.*, p. 12.

4. *Ibid.*, pp. 12, 15.

CHAPTER TWO

THE HOUR OF DEATH

SAINT SILOUAN THE ATHONITE says: 'Do not murmur, O children of God, because you find life difficult. Only wrestle with sin . . .',[1] and truly, our life is hard, because we seek a way of redeeming it from the curse of death.

Our sojourn on this earth is time given for us to learn how to die, but unfortunately, nothing we are taught in this life enables us to deal with the end. Our generation has learnt to trust in its own intellect, in its own judgment, and this hinders our training for the moment of death – the moment when all our powers will forsake us. Even our wonderful mind, in which we have put all our trust, will abandon us. Will anything be able to help us face the hour of our death without fear, when we will be destitute and beyond human help? Can one learn how to die?

We taste of death each time something distresses us or threatens our life, or crushes us. Such sorrows and difficulties are good opportunities for acquiring a right attitude towards death. Death is a fact of life, but the manner of our death is far less important than the way in which we approach it.

In one of his books, Fr. Sophrony relates the following story. In Paris, where he lived for some time, he had become acquainted with two young sisters. One was very intelligent, a doctor, while the other was simpler, a nurse by profession. The two women, who were nearly the same age, had got married at the same time, and likewise were expecting at the same time. At the time it was customary for expectant mothers to attend classes in pain-free childbirth, and both mothers-to-be did so. The one who was a doctor was familiar with anatomy, and she quickly understood the subject-matter. After a few lessons she said, 'That's enough; I have understood everything and do not need to continue.' The other sister followed the course through to the end. The time came for them both to give birth. From the first birth-pangs, the doctor panicked. She forgot all about anatomy and everything she had learned, and her birth was difficult and painful. Her sister, on the other hand, put no trust in her own intelligence, but brought to mind what she had learned in the classes, put it into practice and gave birth relatively easily. The conclusion we may draw from the story is obvious.

Our death is our birth into eternal life. Our efforts in learning how to pray, how to humble ourselves, how to have confidence, not in ourselves, but in the living God, have but one aim: namely, to train us for the great day of our death. And in which God do we learn to put our trust? 'In God which raiseth the dead' (2 Cor. 1:9). He it is Whom we want to know, and He it is in Whom we want to trust when the time comes, when our bodily powers will have failed us, when we shall be beyond human help. The only thing that will help us then will be the attitude of spirit we have cultivated, whereby we will no longer trust in ourselves but in Christ alone, Who died and rose again, Who is therefore able to raise the dead, for in Him 'death has no more dominion' (Rom. 6:9).

We die, and behold, we live again in Jesus Christ. This transitory life which has been given to us is of great significance: it is our one and only opportunity to struggle to prepare ourselves for the great and holy moment of our encounter with God – the day of our true birth into the heavenly kingdom which cannot be moved (cf. Heb. 12:28). Our entry into eternity is our birthday, and if we wish to celebrate our heavenly birthday honourably and join the festival of the newly-born in heaven, when the evening meal is over, let us bury ourselves in our room, instead of sitting around and chatting pleasantly. Let us rather stand before God according to our strength, mindful of the fearful hour of our death, and let us say, 'Lord, at the hour of my death I will be helpless and unable to pray, and so I beseech Thee, remember me. Now, while I am able, I entreat Thy help in that hour. Be merciful, O good Lord, and at that dreadful hour when my strength shall fail me and I will no longer be able to cry unto Thee, when neither angel nor man will be able to extend a helping hand to me, do Thou Thyself come to my aid and grant me the unspeakable joy of Thy salvation.' Thus, we anticipate the moment of our death in prayer.

This prayer will remain with the Lord, and the Lord, Who is always faithful and does not abandon us, will consider our prayer. This is a great and good exercise in learning how to die. For it is with such thoughts that in the last moments of our life, while our soul departs from our body and all our strength is spent, that we, monks and lay-people alike, should stand before the Lord and implore Him as much as we are able.

Something similar occurs every time we cut off our own will, because our self-will is harmful to us. Thus we learn to set our confidence in the Name of Him in Whom salvation has been granted us, rather than in our own reason or abilities. This, indeed, is a very valuable exercise in that it teaches us to die before we die, so that when finally death comes, we will be able to look upon it, not with fear and confusion, but as a dear friend, a long-awaited kinsman who will now free us from the afflictions and tedium of this life, that we may the more fully enter into eternal life, that form of existence that is both truer and better than anything we have ever known.

There are many who fear death. Some people even forbid us to speak about God and death in their presence. This is a grievous thing because such people fear death because they are unwilling to ponder on the One true God. They invent their own religions (since they must have something to lean on), and create illusory supports. But their false religions cannot save. There is only one true religion in the world, and that is Christianity, which is not the invention of Christians, but has been given to mankind as revelation from on High. The Head of this religion is Christ, the Son of God Who became man, died for us and rose again, taking with Him all those who are united with His Spirit, who believe in His word, and who bear His Holy Name.

Death has no mercy upon those who fear it and hide from it. But death flees from those who pursue it fearlessly and stand before it, remembering God and calling upon Him, beseeching Him to be with them at that hour, so that when at last the moment of death draws near, it may come peacefully and painlessly.

This fear of death is a terrible phenomenon. In our service as priests, we observe that all those who have accepted God's word approach death with faith, and their end is wondrous and glorious, though they may be suffering from a mortal illness. We can say that they have found that for which we beseech the Lord in our prayers and in the hymns of the Church, namely, His grace and His great mercy.

Our training succeeds if we accept the hour of our death as the holiest and greatest moment of our life, having dwelt ceaselessly on this moment in our mind, having prepared our defence beforehand, that our protection for that great day might be secured in advance. Whosoever prays to God daily, with fervour of heart and with tears, asking that He stand by him at the hour of his death, will have all his prayers returned to him as a great blessing and joy at that very moment. And the words, 'Enter into the joy of thy Lord' (Matt. 25:21), will be fulfilled in him.

Scripture does not tell us much about life after death. As humans, we tend to resort to our imagination. The Holy Apostle Paul says that the Lord will come again, and that on the day of His glorious Second Coming, we will be lifted up in the clouds to meet Him. And when we would expect St. Paul to say more about that day, he ends abruptly: 'And so shall we ever be with the Lord' (1 Thess. 4:17). For us, joy, life, and Paradise are to be with Christ. He is our light and our peace.

Prayer is the best preparation for the moment of death, because, through prayer, we stand in the presence of the Lord even in this life. We try to keep our spirit in His presence, by calling upon the Name of Jesus with humility and attention, and we know that His is a dynamic presence. But it often happens that we call upon the Lord, desiring to enter into His presence only to find ourselves unable to do so; it is as if we are beating the air. Then we realise that the fault is in our attitude and that we are calling upon His Name in a manner which is unworthy. We must then bow our head, and bowing our mind even lower, let us say, 'Lord, I sin against Thee, even as I call upon Thy Name. Do Thou teach me Thy humility! Do Thou, O Lord, give me a perceptive mind that I may worthily call upon Thy Holy Name!' And then we begin to sense that the more we humble our spirit before the Lord, the greater the power of the prayer that is given us from on High. Thus, the hour of prayer becomes an exercise in how to enter into the Lord's presence, how to stand before Him, and we learn that our abiding with Him should be strong, active, and luminous.

Let us not fail to humble our spirit. If we acquire this blessed habit, many of our faults will be corrected. For example, the thought may come to mind that we have grieved our brother, and we know that in order to be pleasing to God and to remain in His presence we must be reconciled to the person we have grieved. In order to enter Paradise, one must have a heart as wide as the heavens, a heart that embraces all men. If a heart excludes even just one person, it will not be accepted by the Lord because He will not be able to dwell in it. Prayer, as Fr. Sophrony says, is an endless creation; it is a school that teaches us to remain in the presence of the Lord. This effort to remain with the Lord is an exercise that finally overcomes death, which is why our prayer must be neither superficial nor mechanical. We must unite mind and heart in order to learn true mental prayer, in other words, we must pray with our whole inner being, with all our mind and heart. How can God give ear to our prayer if we do not even agree with the words we are saying? And how can we agree with the words when we do not pay attention to their meaning? If we want God to heed our entreaty, we ourselves must first be totally present in the words we offer up to Him. It is good for our mind to be enthroned in our heart, and as we offer our thoughts to the Lord, our words will be heart-felt, and therefore pronounced attentively, one by one. I am certain that if we resolve to pray like this, then God will be our Teacher. As the Lord Himself says: 'They shall all be taught of God' (John 6:45). The Lord Himself will educate us, granting us to be sensible of His presence in our hearts. And in doing all we can to preserve His presence within us, we soon learn which thoughts to accept and which to reject.

Prayer is a school, and humility is the key to success in this discipline. But it is helpful to know our measure, so as not to draw near to God in a spirit of audacity, keeping in mind the fact that we are essentially nothing before the Lord. We are created beings, fallen, false, and wounded by sin. As such, we can only stand before God with fear: there is no room for boldness or arrogance. If we stand at prayer in humble inclination of heart and spirit, we shall entreat the Lord for such things as are appropriate to our poverty. Let us sincerely ask for the forgiveness of our sins, the dispelling of our ignorance, and for other such humble things. Our spirit will thus be preserved by the humility of our requests, and God will bestow the sense of His presence upon us more abundantly.

Let us be humble. Let us have the certainty of our nothingness before God, knowing that the only thing that makes us truly human is the breath that our God and Creator has breathed into us. In every other respect we are earth, and earth is trodden underfoot. Some of the prayers of the Church emphasise the humility of the body, and indeed, the body should be for us a source of humility inasmuch as it is created of earth and will therefore return to earth. What makes us truly precious is the breath of God, received by us at the time of our creation and at our re-creation in holy baptism. This breath is what makes us the image and likeness of God. Let us have in mind this humble thought of our nothingness, and let us refrain from being full of ourselves, that is, from filling ourselves with vanity, and then there will be space in us for God. This sense of our own nothingness produces the right conditions for us to remain in the presence of God. And the more we become empty of ourselves, that is, the more we humble ourselves before God, the more He fills our heart with His divine grace.

Let us also try to form the habit of denying ourselves. We need not worry about the smallness of our sacrifice. We see that for every small sacrifice we make for the sake of God and our brother, God multiplies His grace in us. But we tend to love ourselves, preferring our own comfort, rather than sacrificing something to God or offering to do something for our brother. But blessed is he who denies himself, for the Lord Himself, when He called His disciples to follow Him, required them to deny themselves (*cf.* Matt. 16:24). To summarise, humility and self-denial become the firm foundations within us, upon which God Himself builds the temple of His Spirit.

In our youth, we rarely think about death. Later, we might ponder it rather intellectually and abstractly, but as the years multiply and the problems of old age begin, we behold the warning-signs of this great event, because they affect our daily life in a tangible manner. In His lovingkindness, the Lord has so designed our life that we might come to our senses and be prepared for death when our time comes.

'Be with me, O Lord, at that dread hour and grant me the joy of salvation,' says Fr. Sophrony in his *Prayer at Daybreak*.[2] In other words, 'Give me, O Lord, at that sacred hour, the joy and the delight of Thy salvation, of my true birth into Thy kingdom.' This was Fr. Sophrony's morning prayer; thus was the approach of his last hour always on his mind, from the first moments of every day. Thus can we too rehearse the hour of our death, so that when it finally comes, we can live it in a truly joyful manner. Indeed, cultivating a disposition of this kind in our prayer is the best spiritual exercise: if we learn to die before death comes to us, then, when the hour of our death is at hand, we will not die, but live eternally with God.

There are many ways of connecting every day of our life with that last day here on earth, but we need inspiration in order to do so. We tend to take everything for granted in our daily life because our nature is inclined to earthly things. Unfortunately, this means that we become accustomed even to Holy Communion and, indeed, to all God's blessings. But the day of our departure for the other world is the one thing we can never get used to. All we can say of it is that it has yet to come, and we can be constantly inspired if, whatever we do, we do it with that last day in mind. For instance,

when we partake of the Holy Mysteries, we can say, 'I thank Thee,
O Lord, that Thou hast enabled me once more to partake of Thy
Body and Thy Blood, but grant that I may be worthy so to do on
that day, the last day of my sojourn on this earth.' To be exact,
every time we partake of the Holy Sacrament should be as it were
the first and last time we do so: as the first time, because we know
that we have not been completely reconciled to God; and as the
last, because we live in hope of undergoing our own personal
Passover into Life, the eternal Pascha. We should therefore relate
each moment of our life to that last day, which is our birthday in
that new and eternal world.

In the Lives of the Saints, we read how God greatly assists
His servants, particularly at those moments when they surrender
themselves into His hands unto death. Just as they reach the
last 'Amen' that is within their strength, God can begin with the
'Blessed be' of His power, and stretches forth His hand to help
them. Similarly, just as we begin to think all hope is lost, the heavens
open, for we have stretched ourselves to the limit of our own righteousness, so that the great Righteousness of God, which is nothing
other than His never-ending Love, can now come to save us.

The much-suffering man of God, Job, surrendered himself
completely to his sufferings, trusting the Lord and trying to
comprehend His righteous judgments, and it was then that God
revealed Himself to him. Job then understood and blessed God,
despising his own righteousness as something poor and false.
Moreover, he said to God, 'Alas that I knew Thee not beforehand,
alas that I suffered not greater things for Thee' (cf. Job 42:3–6),
because he realised that the glory which follows is analogous to
the death before which the man of God surrenders himself.

The same phenomenon is observed in the life of the Holy
Apostle Paul, who says that he suffered a thousand deaths for the
Gospel of Christ. He describes one such event which occurred in
the town of Lystra, where the pagans, goaded by the Jews, beat
him severely, then dragged him half dead outside the city; but
God saved him. Later, he mentions this event in his epistle to the
Corinthians, adding that they reached the point of despairing of

life: 'We were pressed out of measure, above strength, insomuch that we despaired even of life: But we had the sentence of death in ourselves, that we should not trust in ourselves, but in God which raiseth the dead' (2 Cor. 1:8–9). After this lesson, the great Paul never wanted to boast of anything – not even in the awesome and great revelations granted to him, for he knew the danger of pride – but only in the sorrows and deaths that he endured for the Gospel. He knew that the God of the Christians is magnified in the weakness of the faithful, and that the life of the God of the Christians is triumphant in sorrow, weakness and tribulation.

'My strength is made perfect in weakness' (2 Cor. 12:9). These were Christ's words to St. Paul, when the Apostle, who was only human, entreated Him that he might be delivered from a trial which had brought him to the brink of despair. He says that he prayed three times that the Lord spare him, implying by this that he had given himself over to vigils and fasting, praying that he hear the voice of the Lord, or be healed. Christ did not grant him healing, but He spoke to him, saying that His grace was sufficient for him, that His strength was made perfect in his illness. This illness kept him humble so that God's power dwelt in him.

The Apostle to the Gentiles surrendered himself to death daily for the sake of Christ. He himself said, 'As it is written, for Thy sake we are killed all the day long; we are accounted as sheep for the slaughter' (Rom. 8:36). He endured a thousand deaths daily because that was the only way to guard an apostolic heart, a heart full of the Holy Spirit, so that it could preach to the whole world.

How can the grace of an apostolic heart be preserved? In one of his books, Fr. Sophrony says that it is impossible to live as a Christian; one can only die as a Christian, meaning that a person who looks after his own life, his own ease, cannot live the Christian life.[3] In other words, if we are always mindful of death, ready to surrender ourselves in complete self-denial to any manner of death for the sake of the Lord, we attract His grace, and we witness God's miraculous intervention at every moment.

Unfortunately, we do not have the self-denial that begets such grandeur in the apostolic heart, which the Holy Spirit builds up in

the believer when He 'descends and renews us', as we sing during
Matins at Pentecost.

But let us be courageous, consoling one another with genuine
consolation of the truth of God, and let us refuse the comfort
of anything less. It is a difficult thing to offer true comfort to
someone who is facing terminal illness; but to those who can bear
an honest word, we say, 'Prepare for your meeting with the Lord!'
For neither life nor death can be stronger than the grace that God
gives to those who prepare themselves for the hour of their death,
for the great moment of their encounter with their Creator.

St. Paul says that God never allows us to be tempted beyond
our strength (cf. 1 Cor. 10:13). We may be suffering from some
illness and praying to God for healing. But if our request is not
granted, let us know that God can give such grace and power as
will enable us to rise above our illness and, through it, to sense
the joy of the presence and power of God in our hearts, which is
our victory over death. (Recently I read the Book of Acts and one
verse stuck in my mind. As St. Peter was going up to the temple to
pray, a cripple approached him for alms. The Apostle said to him,
'Silver and gold have I none; but, such as I have give I thee: In the
name of Jesus Christ of Nazareth rise up and walk' (Acts 3:6). That
is to say, 'I have no earthly riches, but that which I have I give unto
thee.' How wonderful it is to have nothing else but Christ!)

QUESTIONS AND ANSWERS

Question 1: We are on this journey of life and we know that
there is an end, and as priests we are constantly mindful of it with
the robe that we have on, but is there any specific advice that you
can give us to help the laity in understanding or making them focus
on their daily activities towards that end?

Answer 1: Priesthood is a difficult task, and it is a marvel to
see a priest dying in the same state of inspiration as the one in
which he began. Normally, priests die in states of much less grace,
because all their ministry is to take upon themselves the death of
their people. Whatever a priest gathers when he is alone before

God, he spreads to the people when he is with them. He takes upon himself their death and he gives them his life, the life of God which he receives. But how are we to do this? When we inspire the people to love the salvation of God and to fight against sin, when we give them a word which comes from the eternal kingdom, and when their hearts receive that word, it provokes in them desire for eternal life. In fact, everything we do is done in the hope of regenerating the people. I often say to the faithful who come to our monastery on Sundays: 'Do not burden the priest unnecessarily with the trivialities of this life. Go to them and ask for a word for your salvation and be very attentive to what they tell you, because then you will make them prophets, and your life will be enriched.' I do not have a recipe for that. I remember once, a spiritual father from Cyprus came to our monastery and he said to me, 'I have been made a spiritual father, but I do not know how to deal with the people. Can you please give me some advice?' I said to him, 'There are no recipes for this ministry. When you become a spiritual father it is as if you have been thrown into the ocean. You have to swim and come to shore.' That is to say, you have to cry to God continuously and hope for the best. I always feel pity for priests because I know how difficult this ministry is. We are priests, in other words, we are partakers of the Priesthood of Christ, and if all the reproaches, all darkness, all evil fell upon Christ, threatening to annihilate His life if it were possible, as the Prophet said, the same happens to every priest who partakes of the Priesthood of Christ. This means that the priest has to assume the suffering and difficulties of his people, and to bring to them consolation from above, and give wings to their hope. There is no recipe, only this attitude of wanting to help, to promote Christ in their lives, that Christ be magnified in their lives. And I am sure that there is a great reward for the priest whose ministry is done with fear, because he is on the receiving end of every evil and the attacks of the enemy finally concentrate on him. That is why it is a marvel not to be content with the reality of this present age, and not to abandon the inspiration and the hope we had when we started our ministry. We all started with great fervour, and we must not let that life of the heart die away, or else our hope will be stolen from us. We must rather be like Simeon the Righteous who waited steadfastly until the last moment to receive Christ in his arms, and then said, 'Lord, now lettest thou thy servant depart in peace' (Luke 2:29).

Question 2: You talked briefly about prayer, saying that we should never say our prayers mechanically, that we should descend with our minds into the heart. But we who are in the world, with our busy schedule and life, find ourselves very tired at the end of the day. My personal experience is that I want to say the whole of *Compline* before I go to bed, but sometimes I am so tired that I choose some prayers from *Compline* and try to do what you advised us; but sometimes I feel I need to say all of it and I struggle through it, but sometimes I catch myself just saying the words. So what would you advise? Is there a better way? Somewhere Elder Epiphanios says that the devil is always trying to prevent us from praying. He would come home after his long day of ministry, and he would struggle through the prayers, even saying them mechanically because he wanted to say them. And just one last question which is related to that: When we say 'Lord have mercy' forty times. . . . Often, I hear in the churches and monasteries 'Kyrie eleison! Kyrie eleison! Kyrie eleison. . . . ' What do you suggest?

Answer 2: We all experience this, and especially on Sunday evenings. Sunday is a very heavy day for the priest. I think we all tend to have this problem of praying mechanically, with not much heart. One thing that helps is perseverance, because quantity slowly, slowly brings quality in prayer. As for me, when I cannot pray, I just stop and I say, 'Lord, Thou seest my misery. . . ' And I reprove myself until the reproach brings shame to my heart and I feel that my heart begins to participate a little. Then, I continue and I do better for a little while, then I reproach myself again. Here is something to do when you cannot pray: stop and confess that to God, and reproach yourself before Him with shame, because shame makes the heart participate. When I am like that I do not think about the quantity. I just bring my mind to my heart and I try to speak to God from there, in my own words, until there is some participation of the heart. And then it is easier to continue. There was a monk who used to say that whoever wants to be saved always 'machinates'. Our relationship with God is such an incredible and creative thing! Many times it happens that we are inspired by one thing or another which revives us as we stand before Him.

Question 3: One of the prisoners with whom I work, when dealing with the forty 'Lord have mercies', said that it helped him immensely when he realised that he was saying 'Lord have mercy' for all those who were failing to say it themselves. He said that this brought new meaning to saying this prayer and that now he can't just rip through forty 'Lord have mercies' any more, but he says them with the heart. But the question I want to ask deals with the men at the prison who have no fear of death. Their life has been one of either causing death or seeing death all around them, and many of them even expressed it to me: 'You know, I have absolutely no fear of death!' Do you have a word for them that might get them to think about the day of their death?

Answer 3: We said that death becomes a Gospel of life when we confront it properly. In general, every contact with eternity has one of two effects. If man has the right attitude, he benefits; if he has the wrong attitude, he gets completely lost. For example, I read in the *Philokalia* that when the sun shines, it warms everything: when the sun warms mud, the mud becomes hard and brittle; when the sun warms wax, the wax becomes soft and malleable, and you can fashion anything out of it. With us it is the same. If we have a heart to rightly accept the touch of eternity, then our heart becomes soft, and God can imprint His image on it. Of course, some people blame God for death, but who is man to blame God? The Lord prevails in every judgment, because He showed His infinite love for men in His Son. 'Having loved his own which were in the world, he loved them unto the end,' says the Scripture (John 13:1). But some people remain stuck in their pride and find it easier to accuse God. But we must struggle to find the path of humility. When Jacob wrestled with God all night, he found a way of humbling his heart, and when he had humbled his heart, the Lord appeared to him and he heard His voice saying,

'Thou hast been strong with God, therefore shalt thou be strong with people' (cf. Gen. 32:28). With that certainty he went straight to meet Esau, and Esau felt the change in Jacob, perceiving that he was a bearer of God's blessing, and instead of killing him, he fell on his neck and cried. It is a matter of finding a humble thought that makes us strong with God. Then we can face anything, even the threat of death, as Jacob faced the threat of death at the hands of his brother Esau.

Question 4: Many times lay people call the priest, and you go to their death bed and you think that probably the last time they went to Church was one year before you were even born, and they want you to give them the whole history of the Church in two hours and then to give them Holy Communion. These people have a lot of self-pride and during their life they were strong-willed and nobody could get close to them. Is this situation a sign that they are trying to break their pride, that they have seen the light at the end of the tunnel, or is there a feeling of guilt at the last moment of their life? What is going on in their minds?

Answer 4: What can one do at that moment? Just try to say a consoling word, so that at least in that final moment, they are given a little bit of hope. That moment should not be wasted on lots of earthly things. I remember accompanying a priest who went to see someone who was dying and had all sorts of tubes sticking out of him. That person took off his oxygen mask and said to the priest, 'I want to live one more week so I can go and say, "Thank you" to the elder who saved my daughter's life.' And the priest said to him, 'What are you worrying about? It is so much better up there! That is why nobody ever comes back.' The priest spoke with such simplicity and conviction that I would have liked to go up there myself that very moment.

Question 5 (Bishop Basil): Father Zacharias, you shared with me a vignette from your life. You were put in a situation to console a number of people after a great tragedy. Some of us get upset if we are asked at the last minute to preach a sermon on the Gospel we just heard. But Father Zacharias, a visitor in a church, who had just celebrated the Holy Liturgy and talked, was asked by the pastor of the church to speak a word of consolation to a number of families who had come to the church after an airplane crash, in which all of their loved ones had been killed. And God really used Father Zacharias and gave him a word of consolation for those people. I think it would be helpful for the brothers to hear those words, because so often we work within positions of having to console people after real tragedies, not just someone who is in their nineties and dying a peaceful death, but when one really has to speak a word that would bring consolation to people after a sudden death. Great tragedies are times when people's faith can be challenged. Would you mind sharing what you said with the brothers?

Answer 5: It was about a year ago or maybe more that an aeroplane of a company called Helios crashed just before arriving at Athens, and all the passengers were killed. After some weeks I went to Cyprus. In one of the towns there is a church where I always go because the priest is very nice and generous. He even built two churches in Central Africa with the money he inherited from his father. He is very good; he helps everybody who goes to his church. I was giving a talk at his church and there were many people present. When I finished the talk, this priest said to me, 'You see, there are many people wearing black here, they want a word of consolation because they lost whole families, all their beloved ones, in that aeroplane crash.' I did not know what to say. It was a very difficult moment, because how can you console someone if you yourself have not been through greater suffering than the person you are consoling? If you are consoling someone without having suffered yourself, the words of consolation are clumsy on your lips. That is why we try to inflict at least some voluntary suffering on ourselves if there is no involuntary suffering in our life. We have to make some effort to acquire this dimension in our life. I did not know what to say, but suddenly I remembered two events from my own life. Once I was coming from Greece to England by aeroplane, and half-way through, one of the engines of the plane broke down. The air hostesses were going up and down the corridor, pulling out all the things from the cupboards and throwing them under the seats. They would not tell us what was going on; they just kept on saying, 'Fasten your belts! Fasten your belts!' I smelled something not very pleasant and then I just disengaged; I closed my eyes and I thought to myself, 'Now I must say my last prayer to God. It seems that the moment has come when the mode of my existence will change.' And I started praying as if it were my last prayer. First of all, I thanked God for everything: that He brought me into this life, that He gave me the grace of baptism, the wonderful grace of monasticism and – the greatest grace that there is upon earth – the priesthood. I thanked Him with all my heart for everything He has done in my life from the time I was born, and for having brought me to such a holy man as Fr. Sophrony. I thanked Him for everything that my consciousness could embrace, as if it were my last hour, so as not to depart, if possible, with unthanked-for benefits from Him. Then, having thanked God, I prayed that He would forgive all my sins from my birth up to that moment, whether I remembered them or not, whether I had confessed them or not, because of shame or forgetfulness. Then I prayed that God would console all those who I would leave behind, especially my Elder, Fr. Sophrony, whom I knew would be the saddest of all. It was he who had sent me to Greece to arrange something with Fr. Aemilianos of Simonos Petras. I prayed for all the people with whom I had some link and when I finished, I just closed my eyes saying, 'Lord, please accept me even as I am.' After forty minutes we landed in Thessalonica and I saw through the window, along the corridor, a line of fire engines. They were afraid that the airplane would catch fire at the moment of landing, but, thank God, we were spared! Then we waited for a few hours and another plane came and took us back to England. I went to see Fr. Sophrony and the first thing he said to me was: 'The prayers saved you!' I dread even to think about this!

The other episode from my life that I mentioned to them was linked with my father. He was a peasant, but for his time he was very educated; he had been to an American school and knew English very well. He needed thirty shillings to pass some exam to become a teacher, but his father would not give them to him because he was afraid that he would leave the village and that his land would fall into disuse. He wanted his children to continue his work in the fields. But my father had a passion for knowledge and especially for languages, both Greek and English: anything he knew in Greek, he reckoned he ought to know in English as well. He had a passion for eloquence: whenever he read anything in such a style, he learned it by heart, even if it was a satirical piece in a newspaper. He learned passages from the Scriptures and from the letters of St. Basil the Great, because he found the word of the Saint very powerful. In 1974 the Turks invaded northern Cyprus, and they took all his land. They left him only the house and the garden with the orange trees which remained our main source of income. He was very sad, but there was nothing he could do. After some years of virtual imprisonment in the village, he managed to come away from Cyprus for medical reasons. He came to see us in England and he heard us praying the Jesus Prayer in the services, and with the pain in his heart for everything he had lost, and for the oppressive atmosphere in which he lived, in his own house and village, he adapted the prayer to the need of his spirit, and started praying: 'Lord, Jesus Christ, Son of God, save us from the invaders.' And this became his prayer. After some years, my mother came to the monastery and she said to me, 'If your father is not saved, no one will be saved!' 'What do you mean?' I asked her. She replied, 'He prays the Jesus Prayer for half the night.' Finally the Turks pulled down even the fence around his orchard to go through with their animals. When he saw that – he could not protest or do anything because it would have been too dangerous – he collapsed. He had a heart attack and was taken to the hospital. But two days before that, he was in bed with my mother, and taking her hands, he started kissing them and saying to her, 'Was I worthy that Miltiades, your father, gave me such a soul to be with me all my life?' And he was crying with gratitude, kissing the hands of my mother, she who had been so brave. My mother could not accompany him to the hospital, because she had to look after her own mother who was ninety years old. (The Turks had beaten her and she was spitting blood.) So her sister, my aunt, accompanied him to the hospital. During the two days he was in the hospital she heard him saying continuously, 'Father, into Thy hands I commit my spirit.' The way he was praying had changed and he died praying. They phoned me and I went to Cyprus to perform the funeral service. The Turks allowed me into the village for four hours to bury my father. I was accompanied by two Turkish policemen and two UN soldiers. So, I went and I even addressed the villagers who came to the funeral. I performed the funeral. I ate with the Turkish policemen in my father's house. I even gave them some presents, and I returned to Nicosia. The day after, I came back to England and I had to celebrate the Divine Liturgy at the monastery. All through the Liturgy there was a bell ringing in my heart: 'He is saved. He is saved. He is saved.' I could not stop my tears from flowing and one of our elders, Fr. Symeon, saw me and asked me, 'What is the matter with you today?' I said to him, 'I cannot control myself, I am sorry.' With this information in my heart, that my father was saved, I performed the Divine Liturgy as a memorial service for him. After the death of my father, my mother became a nun in a convent in Cyprus. I have only one sister who is a teacher in Athens; so my mother was alone in Cyprus. She left the village because she was getting too old. Fortunately I had very good friends, monks and nuns, who took care of her. She became a nun and she lived the last years of her life as a monastic. One day, after her death, I was praying for my parents, actually half praying, half thinking, and in my foolishness I asked God, 'Lord, when my father died, You informed me with such a bell ringing in my heart that he is saved. Why didn't You give me the same for my mother?' And I heard a voice in my heart, a strange voice, but convincing and liberating, saying to me, 'Because your father was deprived of everything in this life.' He was deprived of everything, not only because the Turks had taken his land, but he had an infirmity in his right hand which made all the gifts he had useless. He had had a good education for his time, but all those things were useless because of his infirmity.

So I told the parishioners these two events, and I said to them, 'Now let us come back to the people you lost in the plane crash. Those people were in that aeroplane for two hours, unable to do anything. We do not know in what way the grace of baptism in them was revived in those two hours, or what prayers they said to God, or how they ended their lives praying, which would not have happened even if they had lived centuries of comfortable life on earth. We do not know how they ended their lives, but we do know that the grace of baptism was theirs, that they were not godless. They would have seen the danger, and I am sure they died full of prayer, and that their death was full of blessing. We know also from the teachings of our Fathers that God does not judge twice. St. Paul says that if we judge ourselves, we will not be judged, but if we do not do so, then God chastises us so that we do not perish with the world. That is to say, if God allows misfortune to befall us once, that means He is sparing us from misfortune in the next life. Eternal life renders justice and corrects all the injustices of this earthly life. Those people lost their life because of a mistake of the pilot, and I am sure God will render them more in the next life. Maybe they are now feasting in the kingdom of God, and we are left behind, lamenting them because of our ignorance and our earthly mind.' Afterwards, one of the people came up to me and said, 'Thank you. Now I am consoled.'

NOTES

1. *Saint Silouan, op. cit.,* p. 345.

2. *Idem, His Life is Mine*, trans. R. Edmonds (Crestwood, NY: St. Vladimir's Seminary Press, 1977), p. 54; and *On Prayer, op. cit.,* p. 182.

3. *Cf. Saint Silouan, op. cit.,* p. 241.

CHAPTER THREE

THE AWAKENING OF THE HEART
THROUGH FEAR OF GOD

MINDFULNESS OF DEATH is as an encounter with God's living eternity, and it strikes the whole man decisively because it manifests the hell of God's absence from his heart, reveals his spiritual poverty and the barrenness of his mind. This painful experience engenders the fear of God, which begins to surround the heart and alter his way of thinking. Just as mindfulness of death is not a psychological emotion, neither is the divine fear by which it is followed: both are spiritual states and gifts of grace.

Any kind of contact with eternity, especially in the early stages, produces a certain fear in the soul, because eternity is extraneous to man. As we have already mentioned, mindfulness of death provokes charismatic despair, thanks to which man is freed from the attraction of the passions and the created world. Similarly, the fear of God which proceeds from divine illumination awakens man out of his age-old sleep in sin and helps him to return to sobriety.[1] His heart is strengthened with steadfast self-determination to prefer 'the things which are not seen', that is, the 'eternal', to 'the things which are seen', that is, the 'temporal' (cf. 2 Cor. 4:18). Indeed, 'The fear of the Lord is the beginning of wisdom' (Prov. 1:7), and the truth and meaning of this proverb lie precisely in this choice.

Such a wisdom with respect to God and His gifts leads man to enter into a kind of spiritual covenant with Him. He resolves not to surrender to the surrounding corruption and eternal death, determined as he is ever to seek out the Face of the Most High, in his endeavour to fulfil 'that good, and acceptable, and perfect, will of God' (Rom. 12:2). In return for his good resolve, he receives illumination from the Face of Christ, and his heart is quickened.

Enlightened from within by the fear of God, man then acquires knowledge of his true state. He starts to see himself as God sees him. He is convinced that the unacceptable rule of death reigns everywhere, and that within him dwell such darkness of corruption and ignorance, that his spirit suffers torment. He gradually discovers the deceptions and wicked thoughts nestling in his heart, and is tortured at the possibility of his eternal perdition.[2] Although he is not fit to gaze directly upon the source of Light, he is nevertheless lucid enough to be able to assess his plight. Most importantly, he does not despair in the face of his wretchedness, because it is not the result of a psychological analysis, but a quality of awareness operated by grace alone. Moreover, hope inspires him to pour out the content of his heart in prayer, and to work together with God for his cleansing and healing.

Even during these early stages of healing and enlightenment, man's heart apprehends certain truths. He clearly perceives the immense greatness of the gospel calling and the unattainable height of the Lord's commandments, the statutes governing His way. He is equally aware of the extent of his defilement. Constrained by fear lest he transgress the divine precepts, he understands that crucifixion cannot be avoided if he is to enter into the kingdom. The grandeur of his aim and the suffering associated with its realisation increase his fear. Heart and mind are ruled by an anxious concern for his unworthiness before the God of love.[3]

As the Lord showed the perfection of His love 'through sufferings' (Heb. 2:10), likewise His disciple, who desires to enter into the heavenly kingdom, must endure affliction and suffering if his heart is to be cleansed. In his endurance, he becomes aware of the instability of his nature. He proves incapable of steadfastly loving Christ Who 'first loved us' (1 John 4:19). Through experience, he discovers his weakness, and is convinced that 'all men are liars' (Ps. 116:11), because they are not able to keep the commandment of love.[4] This painful discovery intensifies his divine fear and this crushes and humbles his heart, making it receptive to the love of God.

The fear of God works differently in man's heart, depending on the various stages of spiritual life. At first, it grants him the wisdom that prefers eternal blessings, as well as the inspiration to seek them out. Then it brings him to knowledge of the weakness of his nature, and he thereby learns to preserve the grace of God.

The place of the deep heart is concealed by vanity.[5] The fear of God is therefore essential, because it teaches man 'not to think of himself more highly than he ought to think' (Rom. 12:3), but to keep the sensation of God alive in his heart with humility. Finally, when Christ's great love increases in the heart, then divine fear acts as a safeguard. It imparts a perfect attitude of humility – a profound sense of man's unworthiness before such a God, a God of love such as Christ. Humble gratitude then unceasingly attracts an ever greater fullness of divine love, until the greatest wonder in the history of the world takes place: 'God united in one with man.'[6]

Man, then, can only love in accordance with the measure of his fear of God. In this he resembles the Cherubim, who try to surpass each other in godly fear, that they might love the Lord the more, with all their being. Both fear and love should accompany man during the whole course of his life, for they preserve in him the kind of heart that is pleasing to God, and in which the Spirit of the Lord can find rest.

In a certain way, the fear of God is natural in the man who has not tasted of divine grace. Though he does not know the magnitude of the Lord's humility, meekness and love, he is nonetheless fearful of offending against His holiness. But if mind and heart are caught up into the light-filled expanses of Heaven, man returns from the feast of divine love to daily reality, and again he will live in divine fear with the thought: 'Will He Who has withdrawn ever return?'[7]

Where he once feared because he was not acquainted with the Lord's mercy, he now knows the great condescension of God's compassion, and he is fearful and contrite because God has departed, leaving an unbearable emptiness. This is the beginning of the perfect fear of the righteous. The saints are earthly inhabitants of Heaven who are seers of the Divine Light, having been liberated from the fear of death. But in their wisdom they fear excessive boldness knowing that contrition alone enables them to remain steadfast as they stand before the Lord. The humility of perfect fear keeps safe God's gift and seals the heart with spiritual knowledge.

Divine fear must possess the believer's soul as he follows the Lord, for it precedes the love that is given at each degree of the spiritual ascent and always follows as an even deeper humility. And when finally man is counted worthy of beholding the Face of the Lord, as he comes before Him, he is, as ever, inspired by this twofold and sane feeling – fear and love. He fears because the Lord is the Creator of all, Whose holiness he cannot attain. He loves, because he senses that God is a merciful Father, Who descends from the height of His glory to dwell in his heart.[8] Perfect love like this casts out imperfect fear, which 'has torment' as John, the great disciple of love, testifies (1 John 4:18).

We can see, therefore, that divine fear awakens the heart of man, builds it up and perfects it with divine love, so that it may receive the invaluable wealth of the knowledge and wisdom of God. Unless his heart has been begotten anew, man is 'vain in his imaginations' (cf. Rom. 1:21), and is in fact disinclined to acquire wisdom (cf. Prov. 17:16).

No matter how pure may be the motives of a man's happy disposition, the fear of God advises him to exercise prudence in accordance with His word: 'Serve the Lord with fear, and rejoice with trembling' (Ps. 2:11). Walking wisely upon earth in the fear of God, he perfects holiness day by day, and receives God's inheritance according to His unfailing promise: 'Thou hast given me the heritage of those that fear thy name' (Ps. 61:5).

Even during the great moments of his visitation and exaltation by the grace of God, man learns discretion, restraining his enthusiasm by humbly preserving the fear of God. Thus is he untainted by human daring as he walks in the good pleasure of God's visitation. 'To this man will I look, even to him that is poor and of a contrite spirit, and trembleth at my word,' says the Lord (Isa. 66:2). St. John of Sinai, who recommends prudence during those great moments when man is visited by the grace of God, says the following: 'Do not be bold, even though you may have attained purity; but rather approach with great humility, and you will receive still more boldness.'[9] Unfortunately, when ignorance and arrogance prevail in a person, the gifts of the Holy Spirit become a dangerous weapon.

NOTES

1. Cf. *We Shall See Him As He Is, op. cit.,* p. 21.

2. Cf. *On Prayer, op. cit.,* p. 9.

3. *Ibid.,* p. 117.

4. *Saint Silouan, op. cit.,* p. 241.

5. Cf. *On Prayer, op. cit.,* p. 11.

6. *Ibid.,* p. 103.

7. Cf. *ibid.,* pp. 13, 103; and *Saint Silouan, op. cit.,* p. 502.

8. See *Saint Silouan, op. cit.,* pp. 177–178, 296.

9. St. John Climacus, *The Ladder of Divine Ascent,* trans. Lazarus Moore, Step 28:12 (London: Faber and Faber, 1959), p. 252.

CHAPTER FOUR

THE AWAKENING OF THE HEART THROUGH BEARING SHAME IN THE SACRAMENT OF CONFESSION

THE FIRST-CREATED MAN AND WOMAN in Paradise 'were both naked ... and were not ashamed' (Gen. 2:25). They wore garments of incorruption and their spirit was directed towards God, their Archetype. But when Adam turned his gaze to the created world and subsequently transgressed God's commandment, he was stripped of the luminous garment of divine breath. The eyes of them both were opened, and they knew that they were naked; and they sewed fig leaves together, and made themselves aprons (Gen. 3:7). Shame entered their lives and they lost their spiritual honour. The presence of the beneficent God had become intolerable for them, so they 'hid themselves from the presence of the Lord God' (Gen. 3:8). Man's withdrawal from God and his alienation from divine life reached the point of his coming to resemble beasts without understanding (*cf.* Ps. 49:12), and in his hardened heart he said, 'There is no God' (Ps. 14:1).

After Adam's fall, man's nature was mortally wounded, even in Paradise. He became subject to corruption and death. And this is why Christ came to heal the sickness of human nature. He came humbly as a man, took our shame upon Himself and, by His Resurrection, clothed us anew in the holy and undefiled garment of His glory, without any 'spot or wrinkle' (Eph. 5:27). He did not leave us even the slightest trace of shame, since, as Scripture says, all 'the reproaches of them that reproached Him fell on Him' (cf. Rom. 15:3).

In his great desire for our healing and salvation, Christ did not spare Himself. 'For the joy that was set before him he endured the cross, despising the shame' (Heb. 12:2). In other words, by enduring the shame of the Cross, Christ wiped away our shame and saved us. He traced His humble path upon earth, so that anyone who follows it is healed entirely, wherefore the Lord Himself calls to repentance all who have sinned and are sick (Matt. 9:12). Therefore, repentance as a means of healing and salvation is linked inseparably to the way of the Lord, and this is a way that willingly accepts shame.

But if he would repent and be healed from sin, man must first discover his sin. When he is far from God, he is in darkness and cannot comprehend how far he has fallen. However, when he receives a word from God with faith in Christ, at the same time he receives in his heart the heavenly fire of divine grace. He is enlightened and acquires a new vision. The effect of this vision is twofold. On the one hand, the fire of grace forms in the heart of the believer the heavenly image of the Word Who created him. On the other hand, the spiritual poverty and the abyss of darkness, in which fallen man finds himself, are revealed. This vision is a wonderful gift from heaven and does not cease to inspire man to ever-increasing repentance. It produces in him a deep need to throw away 'all filthiness and superfluity of naughtiness' (Jas. 1:21) and return in repentance to his Father's house in heaven.

There is, however, a very great obstacle to enlightenment and the twofold vision mentioned above, namely, pride. Pride turns the heart to stone and so dulls the soul's spiritual vision that it cannot perceive the metaphysical 'substance' of sin and its all-pervasiveness. For whosoever is proud cannot love. Pride isolates man within himself and seduces him with the delights of luciferic self-deification. This gives way to a depressing emptiness, and he becomes a captive of hell, and even of madness. He is now so tyrannised by the force of the passion of pride that his only escape appears to lie in the world around him. As he seeks to fill this inner emptiness, he is immersed in ever deeper distortion and destruction, and soon becomes capable of committing any crime or sin.[1]

In this tragic state, man is confronted by a dilemma: either he hides himself 'from the presence of the Lord God' (cf. Gen. 3:8) and 'dies in his sins' (cf. John 8:24), refusing the burden of shame for his sinfulness, or he thrusts aside the corrupt reasoning he uses to justify his fall, and accepts Christ's call to repentance (cf. Matt. 4:17).[2] This acceptance of the word of the Lord, we have already said, brings enlightenment and a twofold vision and perception. On the one hand is Christ's blameless love and holiness, and on the other, the horrific gloom of sin and the deception of the passions.

Such illumination by grace not only brings the soul to contemplation, but also imparts the courage needed to make the leap of confession (cf. 1 John 1:9). The Lord says, 'Whosoever shall confess me before men, him will I confess also before my Father which is in heaven' (Matt. 10:32). However, He also warns: 'Whosoever shall be ashamed of me and of my words in this adulterous and sinful generation; of him also shall the Son of man be ashamed, when he cometh in the glory of his Father' (Mark 8:38). In other words, whoever is ashamed to receive Christ as his crucified God and Saviour, and the word of the Cross, the Gospel of Christ as the power of God 'unto salvation to everyone that believeth' (Rom. 1:16), him also will Christ be ashamed to receive on the day of His glorious Second Coming.

These words of the Lord make it clear that confession and the taking up of the Cross of Christ, in a world which 'lieth in wickedness' (1 John 5:19), are accompanied by shame, even as they carry great power, being the means to eternal salvation. By calling man to confess Him, Christ honours him, and makes him equal to Himself. But if man denies Him, then He, in His turn, will deny man. Although this may seem severe, it is also very lenient. Let us not forget that man is the servant of Christ, Who is Lord of all. The severity of the judgment inspires us with fear, that we may be spared the shame of condemnation and perdition. On the other hand, it is lenient in that it begets in us the shame of gratitude in response to the great gift of salvation, and having thus been granted a sense of how undeserving we are of such an honour, we are equally spared the terrible shame of ingratitude. In other words, the shame and reproach which a person endures by bearing Christ's Cross lead to his being acknowledged by the Lord and, in the kingdom of His Father and in the presence of His holy angels, such shame is transformed into the grace of sonship and the power of life indestructible.

When the believer becomes aware of his iniquity, he no longer does anything to conceal it, but he will confess his iniquity to the Lord against himself (*cf.* Ps. 32:5 Lxx). And the Lord forgives the ungodliness of his heart and renews him with the grace of eternal salvation in return for the shame he bears in the act of repentance. The deeper the shame with which he reveals his sins in the sacrament of confession, the greater the power and grace he receives for his regeneration.

The presence of shame in the mystery of confession is not only healthy and normal, but also confirms that repentance is offered from the heart – that it is voluntary and deeply humble. Whoever truly repents and confesses his transgressions takes full responsibility for them, without justifying himself as Adam did in Paradise. He does not blame God or his neighbour. Instead, he endures the shame of his sins with humility and courage. This act of devotion heals man by removing the malignant tumour of his pride. He is granted humility, which attracts God's healing grace still more, according to the word of Scripture: 'God resisteth the proud, and giveth grace to the humble' (Prov. 3:34; 1 Pet. 5:5).

How extraordinary it is that shame should, by the grace of God, be a source of power whereby man overcomes the passions and sin! But let us consider the way in which man co-operates in this mystery which pulls him out of the deathly swamp of sin, and back onto the path of life.

The Gospel account of Zacchaeus' encounter with Jesus throws a great deal of light on our subject (Luke 19:1–10). This notable and influential man, a tax-collector of ill-gotten wealth, was overcome by the desire to see who Jesus was. But his desire was frustrated by the density of the crowd for he was of small

stature. Zacchaeus, however, was so eager that he thought nothing
of becoming a laughing-stock to the crowd. Because he was willing
to accept whatever shame might come his way, he took courage,
and climbed up into a sycamore tree so that he would be able to
see Jesus. The Lord drew near, and He noticed Zacchaeus. Then
He called him down from the tree so that He could meet him. He
even gave him the honour of visiting his house and staying with
him. And the result of this visit was truly marvellous: Zacchaeus
who had despised his standing with the crowd was put right. All
his former iniquities were made good, and his debts were restored
'fourfold' in righteousness. Christ our God and Saviour declared:
'Salvation is come to this house.'

But how did this great miracle come to pass? Whence came
such power as could make of an unjust tax-collector a righteous
man in whom the good pleasure of God found repose, and in
whose house the peace of Jesus suddenly reigned? The matter
is very simple: Zacchaeus was indifferent to the crowd's good
opinion and willingly bore shame for Christ's sake. And this is
precisely why the Lord noticed him; in Zacchaeus, He saw a
spiritual kinship with Himself. The Lord Jesus Himself was on His
way to Jerusalem to bear reproach and suffering for the salvation
of the world. He was journeying towards the Cross of shame; and
Zacchaeus, in a prophetic way, put himself in the way of Christ
and therefore endured shame. His desire for salvation drew the
Lord to him not only as a fellow-traveller, but also as a guest at his
table. And the Lord's visit did indeed bring peace and the grace
of salvation to his house. Above all, however, it enlarged his heart
'fourfold' – and this turned his life around. The 'fourfold' nature of
his conversion signifies Zacchaeus' assimilation into the mystery
of the depth, the height, the length and breadth of the Cross of
Christ (cf. Eph. 3:18). In other words, by putting himself in the way
of the Lord, that is, the way of shame for the sake of salvation,
Zacchaeus' heart underwent a fourfold enlargement, meaning that
he was reborn unto the boundlessness of eternal life. The parables
of the Publican and the Pharisee, and that of the Prodigal Son also
provide further examples of this path of self-abasement.

The righteous of the Old Testament were acquainted prophetically with this aspect of the mystery of the Cross. When, for example, Josiah, the young and just king of Israel, read the Book of the Law for the first time, he was greatly perplexed and 'rent his clothes' (2 Kgs. 22:11). For he now perceived the apostasy of the children of Israel from the way of their fathers, and God's imminent wrath upon them. So he sent representatives to the Prophetess Huldah to ascertain the will of the Lord both for himself and for his people. The righteous one prophesied the coming of evils and the wrath of God upon this rebellious people. As for the king, she said that the Lord had forgiven him because he had believed in the words of the Book of the Law. 'His heart was ashamed and he humbled himself before the Lord . . . and wept' (2 Kgs. 22:19 Lxx), and for this he was to be spared the evils which would come to pass, and would go to his grave in peace and be united with his fathers. Thus, the king was preserved through the deep shame of his heart, and justified before the judgment of the Lord (cf. 2 Chr. 34:27).

In His desire for our salvation, Christ did not spare Himself in the slightest. As the Scriptures say, 'The reproaches of them that reproached Him fell on Him' (cf. Rom. 15:3), and that this took place 'without the camp' (Heb. 13:13). In other words, the reproach endured by God the Saviour for our salvation could not have been more complete. Likewise, when, in confession, we bear a small measure of the reproach He bore for our sins, we then forsake the 'camp' of this world – its favourable opinion and its spirit – and we 'offer the sacrifice of praise to God continually' (Heb. 13:15). In offering up thanksgiving to the Author of his salvation, the believer sets himself in the way of the Lord so as to meet the Lord Who is Himself the Way, Who is the gracious Fellow-Traveller of them that repent, and Who imparts His grace to man and renews his life.

The Fathers say that the man who voluntarily ascribes blame to himself runs towards Christ's Passion. The Good Thief is the best example of this: his condemnation of himself worked the transformation of his own cross into Christ's Cross, and he was saved that very day. Genuine condemnation of oneself renders only glory to God, putting the blame where it belongs, that is, on fallen man: 'Let God be true, but every man a liar' (Rom. 3:4). The heart of him who condemns himself is filled with gratitude, for he is now truly aware of the truth that 'while we were yet sinners, Christ died for us' (Rom. 5:8).

Before repentance, man's natural powers are directed towards the earth whence he was fashioned. His heart is hard, his mind dispersed in its intercourse with the created world. He is empty within himself, and his true purpose is frustrated, as he journeys towards the abyss of nothingness. But if he repents and confesses in humility, he will discover contrition in his heart. His contrition deeply pains him, because he beholds the ugliness of the fall. But this pain and the shame that comes with the acknowledgement of sin till the fallow soil of the heart, uprooting from it the passions of dishonour. The powers of the soul are healed and unified for the fulfilment of the commandment to love God, and for the worship of the Lord 'in spirit and in truth' (John 4:24). As he stands before the Lord in awe and love, man then receives grace which so enlarges his heart that it embraces the whole race of men as he intercedes before God for the salvation of the whole world. By fulfilling the two great commandments of love for God and his neighbour, man lays the foundations of God's temple, that the Spirit of God might take up His abode in him. (To bear shame for Christ's sake is considered by God as a sacrifice, as gratitude towards Him Who saved us by the Cross of shame. And for that gratitude He comes to us and imparts His life to us. Indeed, our souls are redeemed through this sacrifice of shame, and when I see people confessing truly and in shame, I want to hide myself under the earth. I feel myself all the more humbled, because I know that in their hour of remorse and shame, the hand of God rests upon them and all heaven is on their side. These people are given an abundance of grace for their sincere and humble confession, and they are truly regenerated.)

QUESTIONS AND ANSWERS

Question 1: Is there anything that we can specifically do for ourselves, and to encourage our parishioners to prepare in such a way that their confession is more efficacious and more able to bring salvation to them?

Answer 1: If the people understand why this shame is converted into strength against sin and the passions, then they take courage in confession, and they verify this truth by experience. Once I spoke at a meeting of the spiritual fathers in Limassol, Cyprus, and the title of my talk was 'The Transformation of Shame into Power against the Passions in the Sacrament of Confession'. I spoke extensively about this matter and I remember that afterwards someone said to me, 'Now I want to confess!' Of course, we all have difficulty confessing; it is not an easy thing. I am sixty years old and every time I confess, I find it difficult. I have to go against my whole being. But what deliverance I feel when it is over and done with! It is difficult for all of us, but it is well worth it, because there is such grace and liberty afterwards!

Question 2: We have people who come to us for the sacrament of confession; you see them crying, they are humbled and so forth, but they come back again, again, again and again. And you get just full of 'again'. What would be your advice for me as a priest to meet a challenge like that?

Answer 2: There are different practices. I know that some spiritual fathers stop people coming to them when they see that it is fruitless, and they say to them, 'Find someone else; I cannot do this any more.' We all have such cases. But we can also labour over and over again with a word of consolation. And the moment comes when people are struck in their heart by a sense of dishonour and real shame, and they start making progress. We should not forget that the ministry of the priest is one of consolation. In the Old Testament, God says through His Prophet Isaiah, 'Priests, console my people' (*cf.* Isa. 61:1–2). I think if we are patient and we console them, and explain the matter to them, they themselves will come to a point when they feel that they must either make more effort and overcome their problem, or stop coming to us. But on our part, there must always be an effort to instruct, to console, and also to warn. Fr. Sophrony rarely admonished us; but if he perceived pride in us, then his words were very soft but they could crush bones. With everything else he was very indulgent, but he knew that pride is the beginning of the end, and that everything would be lost if he did not correct us. He did that to me twice – how cleansed I felt afterwards! What a comfort and ease in prayer I had after that – it was a really thorough washing! There are many practices. If I went by the criteria of the Greek spiritual fathers, I think I would surely be lost. They are stricter – perhaps not all of them, but in general. Here in the West, though, because of the circumstances of life, and the difficulty of the conditions in which people live and the world that surrounds them, we have to be more indulgent and patient. But it is good to know the rules of the Church, for example, that a certain sin is punished by a two-year exclusion from Holy Communion. Nobody can apply these rules literally anymore, but it is very important that we know them, because they reflect the magnitude of the soul's deadening when certain kinds of sin have been committed. The time can, of course, be shortened in any case, depending on the repentance of the person, and on the disposition and willingness of the priest to co-operate with that person. Everything can be accelerated if the priest works together with the penitent and prays for him. I now realise that when we priests pray for ourselves, God does not listen to us, He can be as deaf as I am, but when we pray for other people He responds very quickly, which shows that this is the true nature of our ministry. It is very important and very valuable that we pray for the people and be attentive to them. If the spiritual father is willing to work alongside someone who repents, the healing process is accelerated enormously. But there are many factors. In physics, there are various formulas for physical laws; constants are introduced so that under certain conditions the formula works out in one way, and under other conditions, in another way. It is the same with spiritual phenomena, just that there are other constants to bear in mind such as the willingness and the care of the priest, and these are very important.

Question 3: We have many people who repeatedly continue to come back to us, confessing the same sin over and over again. My question is, 'Who is failing?' Are they or are we? Are we really not able to read their spiritual problem, or the reason or cause for the failing? Why do people come back who are obviously not reconciled? They do not have victory through confession and they keep coming back with the same thing.

Answer 3: It is not that they are not reconciled, but 'old habits die hard', as we say in English, and certain wounds take time to heal. I think that if they are even a little bit serious about the matter, it helps, even though they might fall back. It is like when we weed the fields: we take out the weeds and they come up again, but it is better to do it regularly than to leave the weeds to drown the wheat. They may not be as serious as we want and expect them to be, but there is something in them that makes them come back to us again and again, and I am sure that God accepts even that. Forgive me for repeating myself, but we must remember that as priests we should provide comfort for the people of God. Since the times of the Old Testament to the present that was the task of the priest. I remember I had a friend who was a student, and he had in mind to become a priest. He went to ask an old Russian sage what is needed to be a priest. That wise man said to him very simply: 'Two things: to love God and to love the people.'

Question 4: Can you describe briefly the difference between shame and humility?

Answer 4: I think that shame precedes humility and imparts humility, especially if it is a matter of obedience to God's word and commandment. There is no confusion. We are not doing anything for psychological reasons; we want to be reconciled with God Himself; we want to demolish the 'wall of partition' (Eph. 2:14) between God and us. King Josiah, whom we mentioned before, was saved because of the shame he felt in his heart; all the people were to be punished except him. In other words, shame precedes humility because it engages the heart, humbles the heart, and attracts grace which justifies.

Question 5: Most of the penitents whose confessions I hear begin with a statement of their sin, and then follows the expression that they will 'try harder'. What words can you give us to help us to turn the person away from his own will – 'to try harder' – and to trust in the mercy and the love of God instead?

Answer 5: I think that it is not bad that they have this thought to try harder, because all things in our Christian life are a co-operation of the divine and human factor. The divine factor is infinitely great and the human factor is infinitely small; but even so, the divine factor can do nothing without the contribution of the human factor. So, tell them that it is good that they want to try harder, but that is infinitesimally small. They have to implore God and humble themselves to attract to their side the infinitely great factor of the divine mercy.

Question 6: You spoke about the priesthood as a ministry of consolation, but I am wondering particularly, in the sacrament of confession, how do you walk that fine line between consoling and yet not minimizing the shame, not reducing the shame and the power that the penitent people can gain from that?

Answer 6: Very good question! Once Fr. Sophrony said to me, 'The work of a spiritual father is thankless if he has to push people; but it becomes a pleasure and a joy when people are inspired. Then he has rather to moderate their zeal, which is much easier than stirring up zeal in them.' Therefore, if you see that the people who come to confession are full of shame, contrition and are broken, of course you cannot do anything else but console. That is how God deals with us. But if you see that they are hardened, then you could say a serious word with the hope that, maybe, it will touch their hearts. It depends, but if someone comes and he is contrite, accusing himself before God, he is already justified by God, and I cannot but justify him myself by saying a good and encouraging word to him. However, if someone comes to me and says, 'Eh! Nothing serious, Father, the usual things . . .', shrugging his shoulders, not saying much and acting as if sin were natural, then I have to say something, gently warning him that his heart is in danger of becoming dead, hard and unable to receive God's salvation. There are no recipes; at that moment, you must have one ear towards heaven and the other towards the person in front of you, and ask in prayer to be given a word. And God often surprises us and puts us to shame by how quickly He responds to our prayer, and how words that have never yet occurred to our mind and heart come to us when we perform our ministration in the sacraments.

Question 7: Is it ever appropriate, is there any room or place for a follow-up? If someone comes to you and they confess, and the object of the confession is very serious, is there a time that would be advisable in a situation that you would call them and check to see how they are?

Answer 7: I think so. There are certain things which are very grievous and which we cannot overlook. But we must have three things in mind. First, we must think of our responsibility before God, because we stand before His judgment. Secondly, we also stand before the judgment of the Church, and the Church as a Body has Her rules, Her constitutions. Thirdly, we must have in mind the person of the penitent as well. We are not completely free to decide matters as we would like to help the person to the end, especially if the sin is known by many. In that case, we have to be very prudent because we are not able to speak freely. But you are right, we need a certain length of time before we follow up. For example, if a person comes with grievous falls and wounds, we could say, 'Come back in a month and see me', and see what happens at least within that month. We all have the tendency, when a person comes to confession for the first time, not to ask any questions. I am happy to receive and pray for the person, and I ask no questions, unless there is something grievous and it is known by everybody. If the person comes back later and things have not been amended, then we have to take some precautions. I am not very good with these matters. I am sorry that I have to take the place of the teacher, and I am sure many of you know better than I how to answer these questions; but since you put me here, I speak on your behalf and by your prayers. Please forgive me; I do not want to pretend that I know everything.

Question 8: I do not know how it is in the United Kingdom, following up on what you just talked about, but in the United States there is a degree of legal protection for clergy, the so-called 'seal of confession', but it is assumed that the priest also keeps the seal. So if one would re-contact the person who made the confession under certain circumstances, could he be liable in a court of law for violating that person's integrity and be able to be sued, for example?

Answer 8: We must always be very careful as priests not to transgress the laws of the state. If we cannot keep the laws of the state, which are on a much lower level, how can we keep the laws of God which are sublime? However, oftentimes it happens that we are bound to keep a secret and we do so, but the people themselves do not keep it. We must also bear in mind that if both sides keep the secret, you will have more freedom to let your heart speak, and then there is more benefit and help. Of course, we must be prudent as you said. I know that in America, and now it is coming to Europe as well, wherever there is an unequal relationship the law is very strict. If there is any blame in an unequal relationship, like the one between a professor and a student, or a priest and a parishioner, the law is very strict, because the authority we are given should not be used for destruction, but for help and correction. We cannot do anything about it, but just be prudent.

Question 9: Yesterday you spoke to us about self-condemnation and you said something that was very helpful, that if you have a parishioner who is weak psychologically and therefore unable to condemn himself, it is better to encourage him to praise God and give thanks in gratitude, and that would produce a kind of humility. So the same goal is humility, but the medicine is different, more appropriate for somebody who is weak psychologically. Could you talk to us more about making this distinction between spiritual health – where the remembrance of death, for example, is profitable – versus somebody who is suicidal and psychologically weak, and thinks about death all the time; or between somebody who is spiritually able to bear shame versus somebody whose psychological shame is toxic and destructive to his being?

Answer 9: Let us take the person who threatens to commit suicide. Sometimes people do not actually do it, but they just threaten us. I had such a case, a person who every time he came to confess was saying that he thinks of committing suicide. It was somebody who was staying at the monastery for some time, and in the end I was very alarmed and I ran to Fr. Sophrony. (I used to run to him every time I met some difficulty, because I knew that whatever he told me would be from another world.) Fr. Sophrony perceived through his prayers that this person would not commit suicide but was just forcing his way on me, blackmailing me. Therefore, he advised me: 'Go and tell this person that he can do that if he wants, but not here at the monastery and put a noose around our neck.' I did that, and that person came to his senses and never said it again. But myself, I do not have the discernment to see if someone really intends to kill himself or not; my ministration is half-blind. You have to have prayer such as Fr. Sophrony's to see clearly and proceed in such a way. In other cases, you can help the people by explaining to them, 'Do you want to commit suicide? You are right. There is some truth in what you want to do, there is a part of us that must die – not our whole being, but only our "old self" with his desires, thoughts and mentality.' Warn the person that suicide will destroy him totally, but if he puts to death that part of him that must die, that will even help him and save him. There are certain principles, but no recipes.

NOTES

1. Cf. *We Shall See Him As He Is*, op. cit., p. 30.
2. Cf. *On Prayer*, op. cit., p. 133.

CHAPTER FIVE

THE BUILDING UP OF THE HEART BY VIGILANCE AND PRAYER

A BASIC FACTOR in the building up of the heart and the practice of prayer is vigilance, which greatly assists in directing the mind to the heart, and then to God.[1] Vigilance concentrates the entire man in his effort to abide in God's presence and carry out His commandments.

In the ascetic tradition, vigilance or watchfulness of mind during prayer is essential in the fulfilment of the first great commandment – to love God. It aims to ensure that every movement of the mind and heart is in harmony with the Spirit of God, so that man's return to God may be complete, for our God is a jealous God, Who will not settle for anything less than the whole of a man's heart. That is why the Christian stands before God at the very start of each day: he attunes his whole disposition by stationing his mind in his heart, thereby keeping his thoughts and feelings in the constant presence of the Lord.

One way of maintaining this attitude throughout the day consists in the practice of voluntarily taking blame upon oneself. When man judges himself strictly, he is contrite before the Lord, and his whole mind gathers into his heart. He is then the better disposed to cry to God with all his heart and be justified of Him. This practice firmly establishes the watchfulness of his mind, and thenceforth 'it is not easy for the enemy to cheat his way' into the believer's heart.[2]

During prayer, the believer's attention ought to be accompanied by self-restraint and patience, which is also termed 'prayerful vigilance'. This checks the dispersion of the mind and keeps it undistracted in the work of prayer. Indeed, prayer *per se,* as it has developed within the Orthodox tradition, is itself a form of vigilance, in that it involves the repeated invocation of the Lord's Name in a single sentence: 'Lord, Jesus Christ, Son of God, have mercy upon me.'

The first part of this prayer contains a confession of faith in the divinity of Christ and in the Holy Trinity. The second part, 'have mercy upon me', is the supplication of the one who prays – his acknowledgment of man's fall (in both its universal and personal dimensions), his sinfulness, and his need of redemption. Both parts of the prayer, the confession of faith and the supplication of the penitent, are complementary and give the prayer the fullness of its content.

Initially, this prayer of a single sentence is said aloud. This develops into its silent expression, and finally, by the co-operation of grace, the prayerful mind descends into the deep heart of man where the Name of the Lord finds its rightful dwelling-place. This kind of prayer is therefore known as *noetic* prayer, or prayer of the heart.

The continual invocation of Christ's Name and the mind's attentiveness to the words of the prayer foster a stable prayerful disposition. Prayer gradually becomes man's natural state, the soul's garment, and the natural reaction of the heart relative to every event in the spiritual sphere. In passing, we draw attention to the great significance of such prayer at the hour of death. The work of *noetic* prayer is ultimately a preparation for the heavenly life, and the ascetic therefore looks ahead to the end of his life on earth. He trains himself to forsake every earthly care, that his birth into the heavenly life may be painless and as free from danger as possible.[3]

The mind's descent into the heart is not achieved through artificial techniques connected with the posture of the body or the control of one's breathing. Of course, such means are not necessarily without value and can be used as aids in the early stages of spiritual life, always keeping in mind that the supervision of a spiritual guide and a humble attitude in the learner are indispensable. But when all is said and done, the grace of God alone enables the mind to descend into the heart and enter into union with it.

It is unfortunate that there is widespread confusion, not to mention delusion, in the inexperienced, whereby the Jesus Prayer is thought to be equivalent to *yoga* in Buddhism, or 'transcendental meditation', and other such Eastern exotica. Any similarity, however, is mostly external, and any inner convergence does not rise beyond the natural 'anatomy' of the human soul. The fundamental difference between Christianity and other beliefs and practices lies in the fact that the Jesus Prayer is based on the revelation of the One true living and personal God as Holy Trinity. No other path admits any possibility of a living relationship between God and the person who prays.

Eastern asceticism aims at divesting the mind of all that is relative and transitory, so that man may identify with the impersonal Absolute. This Absolute is believed to be man's original 'nature', which suffered degradation and degeneration by entering a multiform and ever-changing earth-bound life. Ascetic practice like this is, above all, centred upon the self, and is totally dependent on man's will. Its intellectual character betrays the fullness of human nature, in that it takes no account of the heart. Man's main struggle is to return to the anonymous Supra-personal Absolute and to be dissolved in it. He must therefore aspire to efface the soul (*Atman*) in order to be one with this anonymous ocean of the Supra-personal Absolute, and in this lies its basically negative purpose.

In his struggle to divest himself of all suffering and instability connected with transient life, the eastern ascetic immerses himself in the abstract and intellectual sphere of so-called pure Existence, a negative and impersonal sphere in which no vision of God is possible, only man's vision of himself. There is no place for the heart in this practice. Progress in this form of asceticism depends only on one's individual will to succeed. The *Upanishads* do not say anywhere that pride is an obstacle to spiritual progress, or that humility is a virtue. The positive dimension of Christian asceticism, in which self-denial leads to one's clothing with the heavenly man, to the assumption of a supernatural form of life, the Source of which is the One True, Self-revealing God, is obviously and totally absent. Even in its more noble expressions, the self-denial involved in Buddhism is only the insignificant half of the picture. In the mind's desire to return to its merely 'natural' self, it beholds its own nakedness in a 'cloud of divestiture'. But at this point there is a grave risk of obsession with itself, of its marvelling at its own luminous but created beauty, and worshipping the creature more than the Creator (Rom. 1:25). The mind has by now begun to deify or idolise its self and then, according to the words of the Lord, 'the last state of that man is worse than the first' (Matt. 12:45).

Such are the limits of Eastern styles of contemplation, which do not claim to be the contemplation of God, and are in fact man's contemplation of himself. This does not go beyond the boundaries of created being, nor does it draw anywhere near to the Truth of primordial Being, to the uncreated living God Who has revealed Himself to man. This kind of practice may well afford some relaxation or sharpen man's psychological and intellectual functions, yet 'that which is born of the flesh is flesh' (John 3:6) and 'they that are in the flesh cannot please God' (Rom. 8:8).

In order to be authentic, any divestiture of the mind from its passionate attachments to the visible and transitory elements of this life must be linked to the truth about man. When man sees himself as he is in the sight of God, his only response is one of repentance. Such repentance is itself a gift of God, and it generates a certain pain of the heart which not only detaches the mind from corruptible things, but also unites it to the unseen and eternal things of God. In other words, divestiture as an end in itself is only half the matter, and it consists of human effort operating on the level of created being. Christianity, on the other hand, enjoins the ascetic to strive in the hope and expectation that his soul will be clothed, invested, with the grace of God, which leads him into the fullness of the immortal life for which he knows he has been created.

Many admire Buddha and compare him to Christ. Buddha is particularly attractive because of his compassionate understanding of man's condition and his eloquent teaching on freedom from suffering. But the Christian knows that Christ, the Only-begotten Son of God, by His Passion, Cross, Death and Resurrection, willingly and sinlessly entered into the totality of human pain, transforming it into an expression of His perfect love. He thereby healed His creature from the mortal wound inflicted by the ancestral sin, and made it 'a new creation' unto eternal life. Pain of heart is therefore of great value in the practice of prayer, for its presence is a sign that the ascetic is not far from the true and holy path of love for God. If God, through suffering, showed His perfect love for us, similarly, man has the possibility, through suffering, to return his love to God.

Consequently, prayer is a matter of love. Man expresses love through prayer, and if we pray, it is an indication that we love God. If we do not pray, this indicates that we do not love God, for the measure of our prayer is the measure of our love for God. St. Silouan identifies love for God with prayer, and the Holy Fathers say that forgetfulness of God is the greatest of all passions, for it is the only passion that will not be fought by prayer through the Name of God. If we humble ourselves and invoke God's help, trusting in His love, we are given the strength to conquer any passion; but when we are unmindful of God, the enemy is free to slay us.

NOTES

1. 'He who seeks prayer with vigilance, will find prayer', Evagrius Ponticus, *On Prayer,* 149 (PG 79: 1200A).

2. *Cf.* Archimandrite Sophrony, *On Prayer, op. cit.,* p. 153.

3. *Cf. ibid.,* pp. 146–147.

CHAPTER SIX

PRAYER AS INFINITE CREATION

PRAYER IS THE HIGHEST and most noble activity of the human spirit. According to the Fathers, prayer is man's 'mirror of progress' on his journey towards spiritual perfection. Moreover, if we go, as we ought, by the Lord's word that 'all things, whatsoever ye shall ask in prayer, believing, ye shall receive' (Matt. 21: 22), we are convinced that prayer, and above all, prayer in the Name of Jesus Christ (*cf.* John 14:13; 15:7, 16; 16:23) is the surest source of help. Through it, man can obtain everything necessary for his spiritual growth and salvation. For this reason, prayer is as invaluable in each person's life as it is for the sustenance of the world at large.

Prayer is a divine gift that becomes active in the heart through the Spirit of the Lord. Man stands before God in prayer, and God grants him His life-giving breath. He is then so closely united with God, that he mirrors heavenly perfection in his earthly life, reflecting it even as the Spirit of his Creator continues to instruct him. During prayer, he clearly observes the primal truth that man was created in God's image and likeness.

The fruits of prayer are beyond telling. Prayer rekindles one's inspiration, dissolves doubts and fears, and revives the desire for eternal blessings. It comforts the heart with groanings that cannot be uttered, heals the wounds of sin, warms the soul and enlightens the mind. It renders man's spirit sagacious, instilling in him an unrivalled resolve to prefer nothing earthly to the things of heaven, and in every labour of whatever kind and in whichever place to be well-pleasing to God (*cf.* 2 Cor. 5:9), be it in death or in life. Fr. Sophrony calls prayer an ever-new creation[1] that unites the spirit of man with the Spirit of God and heals his nature wounded by sin.

If man had not been created according to God's 'image' for the purpose of life in communion with the Author of his life, then prayer would not only be unnecessary and of no benefit, but also unattainable in practice. God, however, in His bountiful love, desires that man be incorruptible and eternal, and prayer is the most precious and necessary means for the fulfilment and perfection of this glorious purpose.

It is normal that man should turn to God with longing. He is the source and cause of man's being and his Fashioner – indeed, the Lord is the very principle and foundation of the whole man. God, on the other hand, approaches man out of goodness and mercy and quickens him by His presence. We reasonable creatures can find no greater blessedness than this contact with our Creator. Before the fall, this relationship was constant and intimate, luminous and direct, for man beheld the very Face of God, conversing with Him, and he was guided aright by His word alone. Man contemplated God and imitated God, and such was his life of prayer. The fall into sin, however, destroyed man's life-giving communion with God, and he was estranged from the divine glory.

But the Son of God, in His infinite lovingkindness, came 'to dwell with those that had departed from his grace', in order to renew the dialogue he had had with man in Paradise, but which had been severed by reason of Adam's transgression.[2] For Christ is a true Hypostasis, a perfect Divine Person, while man also bears within himself the hypostatic principle, since he is created in Christ's image. Man's extraordinary privilege, therefore, is that of working with God towards his perfection as a person restored. And this is undertaken through prayer, as he stands in the presence of the living God, receiving His creative energy for his renewal and perfection.

Father Sophrony says that the first decisive step in the realm of prayer is made when man receives the grace of mindfulness of death. A strange inner sense lodges in his 'deep heart' and informs his spirit of the utter 'futility of any and every acquisition on earth'.[3] At the same time, the inner eyes of his soul are tormented by a vision of his absolute nothingness, in which his whole being is condemned to annihilation. Everything that his conscience has hitherto embraced, and all that has previously inspired him and given him joy now appears as meaningless, marked by vanity, given over to mortality. In other words, the whole created world proves to be utterly incapable of relieving the soul's deep new-found longing for life eternal. The spirit of such a man somehow develops a certain contempt for things visible, and now longs for those things which are by their very nature invisible and eternal, so that even centuries of blissful living in this world hold no attraction whatever. If he now receives Christ 'who has the everlasting Gospel' (Rev. 14:6) with faith, then the grace of mindfulness of death will inspire him with prayer that conquers the passions and restores him to true life.

True prayer, then, cannot be attained without divine grace. If the true God does not condescend, the one who prays will be unable to commune with God's Spirit. The paths of prayer are intricate and he who prays meets with opposition from many angles. His corruptible body has not the strength to raise itself to the level of the Spirit; his mind is not sufficiently enlightened or inspired to surrender to the Great God and Saviour Who 'raiseth the dead' (2 Cor. 1:9) and thereby leap over the confines of fear, doubt, falsehood and ignorance. Furthermore, his social environment and its proud ethos of self-justification, which is 'abomination in the sight of God' (Luke 16:15), is not conducive to prayer. The spirits of wickedness, moreover, cannot bear the saving work of prayer.[4] For prayer draws the entire created world back from its fall, and accomplishes man's sanctification.

If man is to pray in a way that will both unite him with God and sustain the world, he will need inspiration and energy. We have seen how the grace of mindfulness of death powerfully alters man's perspective on life, and prepares man to turn his whole being towards God in prayer. This is because eternity is knocking at the door of his soul, bearing witness to the unbearable fact that every created thing, being tainted by sin, has been deprived of the glory of God and is therefore devoid of true life. He now sees clearly that he originates from nothing, and that he is nothing outside the good pleasure and kind intention of God. This realisation almost inevitably begets in him a humble disposition, a humble faith in God's revelation, and his soul is prepared for enlightenment by grace. This humble disposition is a most precious foundation which will inspire him to turn in prayer and hope to 'the living God, who is the Saviour of all men, specially of those that believe' (1 Tim. 4:10). At this point, man begins to know the action of the right hand of the Most High. He is enriched in his heart by the illumination of 'the light of the knowledge of the glory of God in the face of Jesus Christ' (2 Cor. 4:6). At first, the light of God illumines man 'unseen and from behind', without his being able to see its source – the Person of Christ. But he is gradually granted faith in Christ's divinity, and he becomes increasingly aware of his spiritual poverty and uselessness, for the divinity of Christ discloses the true nature of sin. Man now perceives the metaphysical dimension of his fall from the blessed and undefiled life 'in the Light proceeding from the Countenance of the Father of all',[5] and his sense of spiritual poverty and sinfulness prepare him further for deeper repentance in prayer.

The grace of mindfulness of death must, however, be cultivated, because it unites man with the personal God of Revelation. As he perceives the magnitude of his fall and begins to dread the consequences of sin, he cleaves to God in fear, and this fear of God humbles his heart in all its depth. The heart has now been discovered and rekindled, and there is new strength in his prayer of repentance. He becomes an expression of the biblical truth about man, who is described as a 'deep heart' (Ps. 64:6) thirsting after that sense of divinity which alone can satisfy his *nous* (*cf.* Prov. 15:14 Lxx).

In their writings, St. Silouan and Fr. Sophrony continually emphasise the importance of such prayer of repentance through which man's renewal and salvation are accomplished. Prayer is salutary because it establishes the harmonious co-operation of man's will with God's will. Man's created energy surrenders to

God's uncreated energy, and his merely human existence is totally transformed by prayer, inasmuch as prayer is the expression of his repentance. In the world around us, nothing helps us in the work of prayer and repentance. Inspiration can only spring from man's consciousness of sin and the sense of his spiritual poverty; both are perceived in the light of his relationship with God, which is founded on man's faith in the divinity of Jesus Christ.

First of all, man becomes aware of his own sin, but he gradually discovers that his fall replicates the original transgression of our forefather Adam, as described in Holy Scripture. Illuminated by the grace of understanding and the witness of the Scriptures regarding man's condition, the penitent begins to discern the design and purpose of man conceived by the Divine counsel 'before the world began' (2 Tim. 1:9; Tit. 1:2).[6] This leads him to distinguish in his heart the image of Christ, in accordance with which he was formed, but from which he fell. He then comes to an awareness of the wider ontological dimensions of his sin – as a crime against the Father's love,[7] a falling away from the pre-eternal Person of the Creator, and as suicide on the level of eternity.[8]

But this consciousness of sin and darkness within himself makes him receptive to divine grace.[9] He now heeds the witness of Sacred History, beginning with the third chapter of Genesis and ending with the Book of Revelation, and thereby gains the ideal perspective from which to begin the task of his repentance, for he understands clearly that to persist in a life of sin would be a matter of the greatest self-delusion and, indeed, a willful failure on his part. In his utter need, he offers prayer to God, and his supplications readily reach the throne of the Most High,[10] Who Himself came down from heaven not to save those 'who trust in themselves that they are righteous' (Luke 18:9) and are consequently deceived (cf. 1 John 1:8), but rather those who are sick (cf. Matt 9:12), that is, those who acknowledge themselves as sinful and who know their great need of healing and salvation. Man gains in substance through such heart-felt prayer. He becomes real, for he confesses the reality of his state, a state which marks every descendant of Adam, and is therefore universal. He speaks the truth before God, and this

attracts the very Spirit of Truth, the Holy Spirit, Who enables the
man who repents to worship God 'in spirit and in truth' (John 4:24),
in a spirit of humility and confession, and in the Holy Spirit, Who
accomplishes the awesome task of his repentance and his total
restoration. His prayer to the Lord is rendered worthy of God,
for he prays in a prophetic spirit: he justifies God and resolutely
condemns his sinful life. His prayer becomes 'the court, the
judgment hall and the tribunal of the Lord before the judgment to
come'.[11] As Fr. Sophrony says, the Lord does not judge twice.[12] The
great Paul says the same: 'If we would judge ourselves, we should not
be judged' (1 Cor. 11:31). Though we know that there shall be a final
judgment, and that all men, whether they will it or not, must come
before the judgment-seat of Christ (cf. Rom. 14:10), man, nevertheless, has the possibility of pre-empting this judgment by voluntarily
condemning himself in his prayer of confession and repentance. He
judges himself by the commandments of God in a humble disposition of self-condemnation. Then the Lord, in accordance with His
sure promise, gives him 'a mouth and wisdom which all his adversaries are not able to gainsay nor resist' (cf. Luke 21:14–15). The grace
of the Holy Spirit is manifested in him, cleansing him from his sins,
justifying him before God and placing him in the way of His Truth.
Let us recall the words of the Evangelist John: 'If we say that we
have no sin, we deceive ourselves, and the truth is not in us. If we
confess our sins, he is faithful and just to forgive us our sins, and
to cleanse us from all unrighteousness' (1 John 1:8–10). This reality
is the essence of the Lord's word to St. Silouan: 'Keep thy mind
in hell and do not despair.'[13] And this is borne out in St. Silouan's
description of his own experience: 'I was thinking to myself, I am
an abomination and deserving of every punishment; but instead of
punishment the Lord gave me the Holy Spirit.'[14] And the presence
of the Holy Spirit looses the bonds of sin, implants a hatred of sin in
the depths of man as a sure sign of his forgiveness, thereby bearing
witness in his soul to his salvation.[15]

Therefore, prayer of repentance makes way for the forgiveness
of sins and prevents the final judgment of God by justifying man
through self-condemnation. But it also brings about the creative

work of his perfection as an hypostasis, which task can only be fulfilled in the acquisition of divine grace. Fr. Sophrony confirms this when he says that human nature can be renewed only by the fire of repentance.[16] Man's renewal is an extremely intricate process by reason of the fall, and its deathly consequences. The very nature of man was undermined: it was divided into parts and this loss of integrity destroyed the harmony of its unity with its hypostatic principle. When the believer struggles to fulfil the commandments, he notices his disorder. He sees that he is not in full possession of his true nature. He has one thing in his mind, desires something else with his heart, and is drawn to yet another thing by his senses. There is no unity in his nature as would allow the fulfilment of the first and great commandment: 'Thou shalt love the Lord thy God with all thy heart, and with all thy soul, and with all thy mind, and with all thy strength' (Mark 12:30). Neither does he reflect the ontological truth of the second commandment, which is similar to the first: 'Thou shalt love thy neighbour as thyself' (Mark 12:31).

As we have mentioned, the grace of mindfulness of death wakes man up from the eternal death of sin and detaches him from every created thing, including his own inner attachments. It inspires in him the sense of an absolute need for God's eternity. At the same time, this grace creates his personal communion with God and with all men, for they are like unto himself. He is also united with the whole of creation, which groans under the same condemnation to death. His thirst for eternal life and his fear of failing to reach the great goal of his existence beget prayer to the Author of life, while fear of perdition renders the spirit contrite and discovers the heart.

Fear of condemnation in the divine court of prayer, concentrates all his thoughts into one single concern, 'not to lose such a God and to stop being unworthy of Him'.[17] And the more contrition one feels as he stands before God in fear, the more fervent will be his prayer of repentance.

In order for this prayer to bear fruit by the grace of repentance, which stems from the Lord's crucifixion and resurrection, man must continually deepen his awareness of his sinfulness. Blaming himself and helped by the grace of the Holy Spirit, he reaches a point of conviction, and feels that he is the worst and lowest of all creatures.[18] And because of his humility, his prayer becomes the more acceptable to God, Who bestows an even greater gift of grace upon him.

Fear and humility prepare the mind of man for crucifixion by the Gospel commandments. Crucified, and hence freed, the mind hands itself over to Christ's call. Man now places himself firmly in Christ's way and abases himself according to the Lord's humble descent. His mind descends into the heart and is united with it, and finds the 'place' of his initiation into the mystery of man's communion with God. It is in this place that the Spirit of the Lord prays, operating the unification of man's whole being.

During its descent and union with the heart, man's mind is refined by God's grace. In the fervour of repentance, he takes his leave of every created thing and frees himself from every attachment, stripping himself of every desire or thought for this temporal existence. The pain caused by his acute sense of sin now concentrates the mind's attention in the heart. As far as the mind stays in the heart in its prayer of repentance, so far does the grace of the Holy Spirit increase the flame of his love for Christ, enlightening his mind through the contemplation of Christ's Countenance. Christ's meek and humble Countenance so strikes the soul that its amazement gives rise to great joy within and the hope of the eventual abolition of its mortality. Thus is man inspired and his spirit elevated from its former contrition.

We spoke above about the crucifixion of the mind, its divestiture from attachments, and finally its descent into the heart. This journey of the human spirit during the time of prayer of repentance is full of pain and diverse sufferings. It is a splendid journey, as Fr. Sophrony says, yet the Lord's word is unchangeable: 'In the world ye shall have tribulation' (John 16:33).[19] Nevertheless, he who prays enjoys great spiritual freedom in his capacity to love the God of his salvation, because the aura of Christ's word prevails throughout the suffering of his consciousness.

The penitent experiences a strong attraction to God which envelops his whole being and imparts to his mind and heart a distinct and fiery thirst for the Lord, and he goes in search of the Holy of Holies.[20] This mighty desire of man to approach God cleanses the heart from every foreign element by its intensity and fervour, rendering it free to direct all its impetus towards the sought-for Lord, towards Him Who is 'the extreme desire of them that love Him'.[21] According to Fr. Sophrony, there is an 'all-embracing reaching up to God in [one's] terrible longing for Him, even to the point of death'.[22]

The longer man remains in prayer, the more the intensity and fervency of his repentance attract the abundant grace of the Holy Spirit. His body is then strengthened by grace to endure further spiritual asceticism, while the very energy of his prayer breaks open his heart so that its darker secrets may be revealed and cleansed. Eventually, every corner of his soul will be illumined, and he will perceive the mystery of the Lord's instruction as the road to his complete renewal. This may be off-putting to those who are proud and estranged from grace, but it comforts and inspires those who have truly given themselves to God in faith, because He knows their inmost, and perhaps inexpressible, desire for union with Him. It therefore follows that the Holy Spirit Himself 'maketh intercession for the saints' with 'groanings [of the heart] which cannot be uttered' (cf. Rom. 8:26–27).

If prayer of repentance is further prolonged, and grace correspondingly accumulates, the heart will continue to be cleansed and enlightened. Unnoticeably yet surely, Christ's word will become the sole law of the existence of the person who truly repents.[23] The keeping of the Lord's commandments, according to Fr. Sophrony's experience, has as its normal consequence 'an extreme reduction of oneself – a self-emptying'.[24] In other words, we are emptied of our self-loving dedication to ourselves in order that the covenant we made with Christ at baptism may be renewed, 'that henceforth we should not serve sin' (Rom. 6:6), and that 'they which live should not henceforth live unto themselves, but unto him which died for them, and rose again' (cf. 2 Cor. 5:15). Intense prayer of repentance, exclusively concerned as it is to be united with Christ 'who loved [us] unto the end' (cf. John 13:1), unifies all the powers of the soul, the movements of the mind and of the heart, so that they may worthily respond to the divine love of the Redeemer.

When the task of prayer of repentance reaches the fullness foreseen and pre-ordained by God, then 'it is time for the Lord to work' (Ps. 119:126). The penitent has now convinced God that he belongs to Him in accordance with the words of the Prophet, 'I am thine, save me' (Ps. 118:94). And the Lord replies, 'Thou art my Son; this day have I begotten thee' (Ps. 2:7). The Lord's response is like a thunderbolt from heaven, which shakes the heart of man to its foundations and strikes his conscience as with divine lightning. In the beginning, the word of the Lord brought the universe into being; now His voice imparts divine power that opens up and quickens the heart of man. The opening up of his heart signifies the healing of his personhood, for he is now spiritually reborn and has been adopted by the Father Who is without beginning.

Fr. Sophrony repeatedly expresses reverent amazement at this 'moment of enlightenment'[25] in which total repentance is met with divine intervention.[26] It is a 'miracle' that takes place 'suddenly' and is 'unlooked for'.[27] We can liken this moment to the Big Bang referred to by contemporary astronomers, or better still, to the moment described at the beginning of the Book of Genesis: 'And God said, Let there be light: and there was light' (Gen. 1:3). At this moment man is often overshadowed by the uncreated Light – in other words, he enters into the living eternity of the kingdom of God.

When, in the work of his repentance, the believer endures the 'fiery trial' of communion in 'Christ's sufferings' (1 Pet. 4:12–13), he passes over the 'dry land' of this age 'until the day dawns, and the day star arises in [his] heart', according to the word of St. Peter, the leader of the Apostles (2 Pet. 1:19). Man then becomes true and he is now committed to the task of his renewal, which he will carry out for the rest of his days. His life expresses the prophetic word of the Psalmist: 'The sun ariseth . . . man goeth forth unto his work and to his labour until the evening' (Ps. 104:22–23). Fr. Sophrony's word concerning the world's current crisis gives great hope: desolation and the tragedy of suffering may well contribute to a vast and widespread spiritual renaissance in a great multitude of souls. The light of this hope is all the brighter in that suffering opens up the way for mighty prayer of supra-cosmic dimensions. Prayer of this kind is worthy of God, and it continually moves man to greater knowledge of God and His action in the heart of man: 'Day unto day uttereth speech, and night unto night sheweth knowledge' (Ps. 19:2). Prayer of this kind becomes a conductor of divine revelation, redeeming the temporal life of man and justifying the world's existence. 'Its [prayer's] going forth is "from the end of the heaven, and its circuit [is] unto the ends of it: and there is nothing hid from the heat thereof". It both warms and rejoices us. It is the channel conveying revelation from on High' (cf. Ps. 19:6).[28]

This great rising of the spiritual Sun in the heart of man is the miracle of his spiritual rebirth, the 'Big Bang' of his renewal. Furthermore, it bestows perfect knowledge of the light of heaven and also of the measure of a true man whose heart is so enlarged that his prayer embraces the ends of the earth and all generations throughout time. Having received the vision of divine Light and the experience of eternity, he puts on the image of the heavenly man, of 'the second man [Who] is the Lord from heaven' (1 Cor. 15:49, 47). At the same time, he recognises that he must put aside the image of the earthly man, his true purpose being to dwell with God, 'in Him, in His eternity'.[29] This is why Fr. Sophrony says, 'I must see Christ "as He Is" in order to confront myself with Him and thus perceive my "deformity"; I cannot know myself unless I have His Holy Image before me.'[30]

Prior to such divine intervention in the spiritual life of man, the ascetic form of repentance must prevail for as long as man struggles to subject his spirit to the judgment of the word of God. Through unrelenting and strict cross-examining of the movements of his heart, he is constantly reminded of the fact that he has not reached the height of the two great commandments and this moves him to greater contrition and repentance. This kind of repentance is characterised by the psychological torment that comes with the acknowledgement of one's transgressions, imperfections, failures and ignorance.[31] After the rising of the spiritual Sun, however, the believer's repentance takes on a firmer, more charismatic character. Henceforward he will no longer take ordinances or authorities as his point of reference, for he now refers in everything to the very Lord of Heaven and Earth, to Whose image he cleaves even as he beholds it in his heart. In this form of repentance, the divine factor is the more prevalent, the transition having been made in man's spirit from the psychological level to the ontological level of divine action. It is no longer man who toils but rather the grace of God which is with him (*cf.* 1 Cor. 15:10).

By this stage, man is taught by God Himself. His consciousness of his sinfulness is all the deeper, because he now compares himself neither with man nor yet angel, but with the Creator and Almighty God. Each action or movement of the heart that lessens or weakens the experience of grace is perceived as a falling away from the love of the God he has encountered. In his effort to preserve grace, his repentance now takes on a particularly ascetic character, in which the practice of ascetic humility prevails, its highest point being when man sees himself as the worst of all. The humility by which man is inspired in this charismatic form of repentance is indescribable. It is of God. Man sees the utterly meek and humble form of Jesus in his heart and surrenders to divine love, and in his prophetic yearning he echoes the words of St. John the Baptist: 'He must increase, but I must decrease' (*cf.* John 3:30). So struck is he with amazement at the form of the Lord that he now knows himself to be truly unworthy of belonging to such a God, Who is exceedingly humble and has loved us unto the end (John 13:1).

The transition from the psychological level to the ontological level of existence, which follows prayer of repentance, is accompanied not only by an outpouring of divine Light, but also by a flood of divine love which opens and enlarges the heart to embrace heaven and earth. Prompted by divine love, man relates to the personal God as hypostasis. He brings all creation before God and intercedes for every human soul. A kind of transformer is implanted in him which, motivated by divine love, enables him to turn every created energy into a spiritual one. In this way, he labours first of all towards his salvation and then towards the salvation of the whole world. The words of the Apostle are then fulfilled: 'All things work together for good to them that love God' (Rom. 8:28). Every energy, of joy or sadness, is transformed into the energy of repentance; sufferings become material for prayer and expressions of love (*cf.* 2 Cor. 7:10; Jas. 5:13).

According to Fr. Sophrony, unless he encounters the living God, man cannot learn the knowledge necessary for the transformation of his psychological states into spiritual experiences, at least, not in any deep ontological sense. Love alone has the power to render every state he experiences in life, be it pleasant or painful, into something that is beneficial and easy to bear. Every such transformation contributes to his recovery of eternity, which itself becomes the actual living content of man according to his development as an hypostasis. Fr. Sophrony maintains that 'all our many-sided experience of life, the whole world-system that contributes to our cognition, must serve to prepare us for a personal encounter with [God].'[32] We meet with the same teaching in embryonic form in the Desert Fathers. They explain that this change is effected by the use of every sensation or energy received from the created world in the turning of one's attention to the remembrance of God. If a man possesses the knowledge which is granted to those who have the mind of Christ, he transmutes the finite earthly energies that assail him into such energy as he can use to intensify his dialogue with God: he 'brings every thought into captivity for obedience to [and love of] Christ' (2 Cor. 10:5). But unless he be educated by the grace of God, man cannot be nourished by the 'solid food' of God-pleasing sufferings, nor can his faculties be trained to discern the righteousness of the Cross, which alone leads to the kingdom of heaven (*cf.* Heb. 5:14). And such training is given by Christ Himself, Who accepted persecution and the smiting of death as the Cup of the Father, to Whom He prayed without turning His attention to those who were crucifying Him. Instead, He entrusted Himself to Him Who judges rightly and prayed: 'Father, forgive them, for they know not what they do' (Luke 23:24).

In repentance on the psychological level, man offers his freedom and his will as a sacrifice to God. God accepts this sacrifice and recompenses man with grace, which enables him to overcome the limitations of his earthly existence and to enter into the stream of His eternity.[33] This ontological change is a revelation to man, and his spirit is captivated by a new depth of prayer, which leads him definitively beyond the narrow prison of this world into the liberty of God's infinity.[34] On the last page of his writings, St. Silouan describes the effects of this revelation with the simplicity that so characterises his authenticity. As he puts it, man is captured by the love of God: 'All day, all night, my soul is taken up with Thee, O Lord. . . . No earthly thing can occupy my thoughts – my soul desires only the Lord.'[35]

The radical event of man's renewal by divine Light and his transition from the psychological to the ontological level of existence does not, however, signify a permanent state in this present life. While it affords true knowledge of God's merciful condescension to man on the one hand, yet, on the other, it brings man's despicable nothingness firmly home to him. The vision of God's eternal holiness floods the soul with hitherto unknown gratitude and strength, but at the same time man is challenged by unbearable horror at his spiritual poverty, for he now knows how grave would be his failure to fulfil his pre-eternal destiny, which is to be united with the God of love for all eternity. The experience of Christ's pure love, which is imparted with the vision of His image, brings a totally different kind of repentance, a fuller repentance which engages the whole of man's being. The light of grace helps man to go deeper into the mystery of his spiritual poverty, and he turns away from himself, shedding bitter tears for his uselessness. He is in complete despair over himself, but at the same time he trusts fully in God, 'who raiseth the dead' (2 Cor. 1:9). Such despair is charismatic for it gives energy and wings to prayer so as to bring the whole of man's being into the sphere of the eternal Spirit. The upward surge of the spirit is also imparted to the body, which so thirsts for the living God. This signifies the sanctification of the body, which is reinforced with grace so as to bear divine love.

The alternation between the two aspects of the vision that we have been describing pushes man to the utmost intensity of repentance. He penetrates in spirit into the eternal design of God the Saviour for His reasonable creatures, and this gives rise to an unbearable longing to overcome the narrow confines of his fallen nature, and to plunge into the unfathomable abyss of the spiritual world. In this spiritual sphere, 'there is nought and no one save the God of love and a vision of His boundlessness'.[36] Man then sees his inner hell in the light of God's holiness and in the burning of His pure love, and this provokes in the soul an irresistible desire to 'break out of the suffocating chains of our Fall' and to be wholly given over to the God Who is the Light of Love.[37]

The spiritual power of this twofold vision establishes and inspires man in his repentance, which is now of ontological, Adamic proportions. Initially, he lives the 'hell' of his personal repentance in order to fulfil the first great commandment – love towards God. To the degree that he assimilates the image and the spirit of the Second Adam, he also discovers his ontological unity with the whole race of mortal men. He now understands Christ's love for the world 'unto the end', and he can affirm how he himself falls short of fulfilling the second commandment – to love his neighbour, that is, all his fellow-men. Just as Christ offered up His own life, so too does he descend into a veritable 'hell of love' in the spirit of Christ, and he offers unwavering repentance on behalf of the whole Adam. According to Fr. Sophrony, the final degree of this repentance, though unattainable upon earth, would lead one into full knowledge of 'the One God in Three Persons and our own immortality'.[38]

Only this twofold vision is strong enough to awaken man from the age-long sleep of sin.[39] It leaves him between the 'hell' of self-knowledge and the abyss of knowledge of God, and thus brings him to a complete knowledge which encompasses all the dimensions of the spiritual world. The momentum of his repentance is powerful enough to 'transport him to unforeseen frontiers, where he experiences a foretaste of divine universality'.[40] If he treads the path of repentance to the end, his spirit will 'know the things of man', and the Holy Spirit, Whom he has now received, will enable him to 'search out the deep things of God' (1 Cor. 2:11). The vision of God's holiness, on the one hand, and man's nothingness, on the other, renders man like unto God. This likeness is powerful beyond measure, and neither on earth nor in heaven can there be an end to it, since Christ is unattainable in the perfection of His love.

QUESTIONS AND ANSWERS

Question 1: Is there a difference between prayer and worship? In other words, when we pray, are we worshipping, and when we worship, are we praying, or can they be different? You also mentioned that, with suffering, we return our love to God. Being Orthodox Christians, are we to understand that we cannot return love to God or fully practise our faith if we are not suffering or if we go through periods of even going so far as to experience luxury?

Answer 1: These are two very big questions. We shall need another talk! Let us take the first one: prayer and worship. Worship is a more general term and an all-embracing life, while prayer is an activity of worship. Worship is more like the exchange of man's life for the life of God, which takes place in the Divine Liturgy, for example. The Divine Liturgy is worship; there is prayer and a whole life there, the life of Christ. In the Holy Eucharist, we accomplish the exchange of our limited and temporal life for the unlimited and infinite life of God. We offer to God a piece of bread and a little wine, but in that bread and wine, we place all our faith, love, humility, expectation of Him, all our life. And we say to God, 'Thine own of thine own, we offer unto Thee in all and for all.' We offer to God all our life, having prepared ourselves to come and stand before Him and do this act. And God does the same: He accepts man's offering and He puts His life – the Holy Spirit – in the gifts, transmaking them into His Body and Blood, in which all the fullness of Divinity is present, and He says to man, 'The Holy things unto the holy.' God accepts our gifts and fills them with His life, and He renders them back to us. Consequently, we could say that worship is a more complete thing. In prayer also, we make that exchange, but it is more unilateral.

Your second question is very difficult. God has shown His love for us by His suffering death for us, and He gives us the possibility, through suffering, to show our love for Him. In this world Christ is suffering, says St. Paul (Acts 26:23), and if we are members of His Body, we cannot be without pain when the Head of this Body bears a crown of thorns. If we understand that, suffering becomes a privilege for those who belong to that Body: the privilege of showing their harmonious unity with the Body. That is why St. Peter says in his Epistle, 'Judgment must begin at the house of God.... And if the righteous scarcely be saved, where shall the ungodly and the sinner appear?' (1 Pet. 4:17). As God delivered his Only-begotten Son to death, so does He deliver His own people, His elect, to suffering, to prove them to be 'His house', that is to say, His dwelling-place, because He lives in them. Thus, if we perceive suffering from this perspective, it becomes a great privilege and honour and the sign of our election by our Heavenly Father to suffer the same judgment that His Son bore in this world, and be delivered unto death too. Death for the sake of God, for the sake of His commandments, is a death that condemns death, just as the death of our Lord condemned and destroyed death. All the saints of God are delivered up to such suffering. Many times, by the providence of God, the Lord allows them to taste of hell – not to be destroyed, but to fathom the mystery of Christ's descent into Hades in order to know *totus Christus* and His path from the Heaven of Heavens to the nethermost parts of the earth. 'Now that he ascended, what is it but that he also descended first into the lower parts of the earth?' says St. Paul in wonder (Eph. 4:9). This is the path of Christ: first, He descended and then He ascended, and all His saints, through suffering, have the privilege of proving themselves to be the house of God and of receiving knowledge of the entire length of the way of Christ. Consequently, when suffering is envisaged in such a way, it is a marvel, a great honour and a supernatural gift. That is why we are not impressed by nice Buddhist theories which try to invent ways of disengaging from suffering, because we have the possibility, through suffering, to become sons of God, to share the victory of the Son of God over death. What is important, as St. Peter says in his epistle, is that we suffer innocently, not in a sinful way (1 Pet. 2:19).

In Nicomedia, there were twenty thousand martyrs heading towards martyrdom. They were all about to suffer death for Christ's sake, but on their way to their martyrdom, one of them tore up a portrait of the emperor. Consequently, the Church did not number him among the martyrs. He had committed a transgression that could be punished by the law of the state, whereas the others were led like sheep to the slaughter, and their martyrdom was recognised as glorious. The one who tore up the portrait was put to death with the others, and probably God received his martyrdom; but because he reacted in a way which betrayed a certain resistance to the evil one, the Church did not count him with the others. Christ says, 'Resist not evil' (Matt. 5:39), and He Himself gave us an example; He was led as a lamb to the slaughter and as a sheep before the shearer, says the Prophet Isaiah (cf. Isa. 53:7), and He was hated without a cause (cf. John 15:25). It is important that we learn the ethos, the manner of life inspired by the Divine Liturgy. We priests begin the Prothesis saying, 'as a sheep He was led to the slaughter and as a lamb before her shearer. In His humiliation was His judgment lifted up.' This is the ethos that the Holy Liturgy inspires; and this is the ethos that conquers death! That is how the Lord overcame death in our place and conquered this world fallen into sin. We must not be attracted by the spirit of this world and take vengeance or fight for our justification, we should rather suffer injustice. As St. Paul says, 'Why do you not rather suffer injustice instead of going to the civil courts?' (cf. 1 Cor. 6:7). He preferred that his disciples suffer injustice than that they fight for their justification, even when they were humanly right. This perfect principle is inspired by the Lord's way. Of course, living in this world, we must do according to our measure in each situation. For us the highest model and reference is what the Lord Himself showed us.

I could say even more if you like in answering the second question. For example, the Mother of God should not have died, according to the tradition of the saints, because she never sinned, not even by a single thought, and whoever does not sin does not die.

Nevertheless, she accepted death but only for three days; then she rose again and was translated to heaven. She went through death so as to follow the path of her Son, so that her death, too, would be a condemnation of death, being an innocent death because of her sinlessness. St. Maximus the Confessor says that those who receive baptism and do not sin after that, should not normally die, not even a physical death. Still, God allows that they die, but their death is a condemnation of death, just as Christ's death was a condemnation of death.

Question 2: We are living in a context where our suffering is really reduced according to how well off we are in this culture. Moreover, in a culture like this, we are told that suffering is to be avoided, to be medicated down and so forth. I thought that maybe you could comment on this.

Answer 2: The culture of this world is to avoid suffering and to create comfort. We all know that, and we are children of this world. But in the Gospel, there is an inverted perspective: all the things that are appreciated by man are an abomination to God. I remember a very beautiful expression of St. Isaac the Syrian, who said that no one ever ascended to heaven with comfort. We all try to avoid pain and suffering, and I do the same. But at least we should know the truth about suffering, to be able to endure it courageously when we cannot avoid it. Then God can give us the grace to rise above it. It is good to know what is true and divinely appreciated by God. We may come to a point in our life when we will apply this theory and then we shall know the veracity of the matter.

I read in the Holy Fathers that God appreciates three things: pure prayer, monastic obedience, and giving thanks when we are threatened by death because of illness, persecution or tribulation. Once I went to the hospital to have an operation. I had to stay there for one week and the thought came to my mind that I had the possibility to try one of those three things. I made the resolution that during all this time I would not say any other prayer but, 'Glory be to Thee, O God, glory be to Thee. I thank Thee for all things.' I prayed for several days in this way, and towards the end of the week, it was so beautiful, comforting and luminous that I was sad to leave the hospital. Thus, the fact that I had read somewhere that giving thanks in illness was pleasing to God was important, because when the time of need came, I knew the theory and I applied it and God came to my help. So, it is good to know what is perfect and appreciated by God. All the truth of the Gospel that we are told and we read about will come in handy at the moment of need and will save us.

If suffering is the sign of our election by God, why do we then pray to be spared from suffering and to have a painless and peaceful end? It is the same with temptations: in the Lord's Prayer, we entreat God not to be led into temptation, but the Holy Apostle James says that when we fall into temptation we should consider it a joy, because we have a chance to prove our fidelity to God (cf. Jas. 1:2, 12). In temptations and sufferings, it is not we who make the plans, we do not choose our cross, but we accept the cross that the all-wise Providence of God allows in our life. God knows how big or small a cross we need. He will give us just that cross which is absolutely right and necessary for us to be disentangled from all our attachments in this transitory life, and to run after Christ with a free heart. Consequently, it is not we who choose; divine providence sets the plan for our life. Of course, we pray to be spared from suffering and to have a peaceful and painless end, because we do not know if we will be able to bear suffering or whether we will become fainthearted. As with temptations, we pray to be spared from afflictions, but if they come, then, in the strength of God's Spirit, we will bear them. Many people arrogantly choose their cross, and they become fainthearted and fall. We remember how the Great and Holy Apostle Peter learned his lesson. If we are faithful in that which is little and we bear it, strength will be added to us to help us bear that which is much and be even more faithful to God.

NOTES

1. *Cf. On Prayer, op. cit.,* Ch.1.

2. *Cf. ibid.,* pp. 110–111.

3. *We Shall See Him As He Is, op. cit.,* p.11.

4. *Cf. On Prayer,* op. cit., p. 12.

5. *Ibid.,* p. 115.

6. *Cf. On Prayer, ibid.,* pp. 26, 57.

7. *Ibid.,* p. 84.

8. *Cf. We Shall See Him As He Is,* op. cit., p. 37.

9. *Ibid.,* p. 26.

10. *Ibid.,* p. 41.

11. St. John Climacus, *The Ladder of Divine Ascent,* op. cit., Step 28:1 (London: Faber and Faber, 1959), p. 250.

12. *On Prayer,* op. cit., p. 52.

13. *Saint Silouan,* op. cit., pp. 208–221.

14. *Ibid.,* p. 435.

15. *Ibid.,* p. 347.

16. *On Prayer,* op. cit., p. 175.

17. *Ibid.,* p. 21.

18. *Ibid.,* p. 157.

19. *We Shall See Him As He Is,* op. cit., p. 222.

20. *Ibid.,* p. 67.

21. Hymn from the *Supplicatory Canon to the Mother of God.*

22. *We Shall See Him As He Is,* op. cit., p. 178.

23. *Ibid.,* p. 229.

24. *Ibid.,* p. 145.

25. *Ibid.,* p. 222.

26. *Ibid.,* pp. 46-47.

27. *On Prayer,* op. cit., p. 128; *We Shall See Him As He Is,* op. cit., pp. 67, 164.

28. *On Prayer, ibid.,* p. 129.

29. *Cf. We Shall See Him As He Is,* op. cit., p. 68.

30. *Ibid.,* p. 59.

31. *Ibid.,* p. 42.

32. *Ibid.*, p. 214.

33. *Cf. ibid.*, p. 152.

34. *Ibid.*, p. 198.

35. *Saint Silouan, op. cit.*, p. 504.

36. *We Shall See Him As He Is, op. cit.*, pp. 44–45.

37. *Ibid.*, p. 22.

38. *Ibid.*, p. 36.

39. *Ibid.*, p. 21.

40. *Ibid.*, p. 88.

CHAPTER SEVEN

THE BUILDING UP OF THE HEART BY THE GRACE OF REPENTANCE

CHRIST'S GOSPEL BEGINS with the words: 'Repent: for the kingdom of heaven is at hand' (Matt. 4:17). These words resume the dialogue between God and man, which was severed in Paradise by the disobedience of our forefathers.[1] But these words are now proclaimed with a new creation in view, a new generation, whose Head is Christ, the Creator Himself. It follows that repentance is the beginning of our turning against sin, so that God's original purpose for man and His creation of man in His image and after His likeness may finally be fulfilled.

There comes a time in man's life when he feels that all the works he has undertaken bear the seed of corruption and are unable to stand before the gaze of the eternal Judge. Such a perception leads to what Fr. Sophrony called 'blessed despair', which, in turn, leads to repentance. This is that same 'godly sorrow [which] worketh repentance to salvation' that the Apostle spoke about (2 Cor. 7:10).

It is said in the life of St. Ambrose of Optina that, shortly before his death, he was asked what rule of prayer he had kept, and the saint replied, 'There is no better rule than the rule of repentance which the publican teaches us: "God be merciful to me, a sinner."' It often happened that, before their death, great saints like St. Sisoes the Great asked God to prolong their life so that they could have more time for repentance. This shows that repentance is not only necessary at the outset, but also in the middle and at the end of one's spiritual life.

Man's first step towards repentance is to sever his ties with the outside world so as to enter his deep heart. The second step is to find the deep heart so that he may be healed by God's grace, and find unity within himself as well as with the whole world.

Christian life begins with faith in Christ and repentance, which are laid down by the Church as conditions for baptism. According to the teaching of the Fathers, man's natural birth of his parents is followed by a second birth which is spiritual, and accomplished by the sacrament of baptism. But there is also a third birth which is accomplished by tears of repentance.[2]

Christian life is not static: it grows and is dynamic. The believer must keep the spirit of repentance even after baptism, so as to make good use of the grace he has received. He does this by keeping God's commandments. According to St. Mark the Ascetic, the Lord is hidden within His commandments.[3] Therefore, by keeping the commandments, the believer is pleasing to his God and Father; he shows that he is a regenerated child of God. He fulfils His will and remains in his Father's house.

According to the Prophet Isaiah, there are two levels of life and thought: divine and human. They are as far from each other as heaven is from earth (Isa. 55:9). By the grace of repentance, man keeps to the divine level – in the vision inspired by the divine commandments. Thus is he preserved and he grows as a child of God.

Repentance is an all-embracing gift because it contains all the virtues. The Holy Abba Ammonas likens a monk's repentance to a fiery circle which encompasses him and protects him from sin. Repentance keeps him in the right thoughts and grants him a right vision, because it frees him from the human way of thinking which is abomination in the sight of God, and orientates him heavenward. Deep repentance can be prompted either by an awareness of one's sins, or the feeling that one cannot live up to the greatness of God's calling. Characteristic examples of both cases can be seen in the chief apostles, Peter and Paul. Remembering their sin, they repented; yet the grace of their repentance revealed God's pre-eternal plan for man to them, and this led them to the fullness of repentance. In other words, they started with personal repentance, and this opened up to them the vision of God's pre-eternal purpose for man.

From its early stages, repentance is accompanied by great consolation. As the fulfilment of a commandment, it carries a reward from God. Repentance is abstention from the dead works of sin and attachment to the living God. It is inspired by faith, which quickens and leads to an abundance of life (cf. John 10:10). It overcomes man's alienation and re-unites him with God, his Archetype.

Thus, repentance in a spirit of faith and humility gives the believer hope that he will not die in his sins. Whoever really repents cannot suffer from morbid despair, because he is consoled. He can only despair of his spiritual poverty, and he lives the grace of this despair alone with the One God. Contrariwise, whoever is sullen in the company of his fellows shows that he is not living his despair alone before God. He burdens his brethren, when he has been commanded to be pleasing to them (cf. Col. 3:15).

Father Sophrony used to stress repentance as a way of life in which one can find one's heart, which is the meeting-place of God and man. Repentance breaks down the walls surrounding the heart. In the early stages, tears are more often than not of a psychological character, as the expression of regret. Yet they are to be valued since they relate to God and recruit man's spiritual powers. (I remember once a young Greek girl told Fr. Sophrony, 'Father, I cry very easily, maybe it is psychological, maybe I am wrong.' Fr. Sophrony replied, 'Let the tears come and turn them into prayer.' That is to say, it does not matter if the tears are psychological, for if we mingle prayer with them, they become spiritual.) Nevertheless, when the heart opens, our weeping is of another kind. Such weeping is like the earthquake of old in the life of the Prophet Elijah. The earthquake is necessary so that the gentle breeze can follow (cf. 1 Kgs. 20:11–12). The rushing mighty wind comes first and makes ready for the coming of the Comforter. The earthquake and the rushing mighty wind are the travail of repentance, which cleanses man's heart from filth and the corruption of death, so that he can receive the incorruptible consolation of the Spirit.

Repentance opens up man's deep heart before God, so that the grace of the Holy Spirit may abide therein. When man receives grace of this kind, he experiences the beginning of his third birth – the birth wherein he works together with God for his regeneration. Man then acquires the state of Christ. In his heart, he receives Christ Who Himself becomes the minister of his salvation. The eyes of his soul are opened, and he sees God and his neighbour in a different way.

The first commandment of love is fulfilled through repentance, because man's whole desire is directed towards God. Repentance unifies all his powers, and he turns towards God with his whole being until he reaches the level of God's great commandment, which is to love God with all one's soul, mind and heart (Matt. 22:37; cf. Deut. 6:5). He begins to see his brother and the whole world as God sees them, and from then on his one desire is 'that all may be saved by Him', as St. Silouan used to say. He longs and prays that the portion of mercy he has obtained may become the lot of all mankind. Thus, man becomes universal, and comes 'unto the measure of the stature of the fulness of Christ' (Eph. 4:13).

Finally, through repentance man becomes true, for he now fully recognises the sinfulness of his fallen nature. As the Apostle and Evangelist John says, 'If we say that we have no sin, we deceive ourselves, and the truth is not in us' (1 John 1:8). But sin is the inheritance and regrettable 'contribution' of every man (cf. Rom. 3:23), because of the cosmic dimensions of its consequences. As soon as the believer perceives his sin, he does not hide it, but confesses his fall before the Face of God. He brings his sin to light and it is wiped away. In this lies the power of the mystery of confession: whosoever repents and confesses his fall before God acknowledges a universal truth, and if there is a time when man is infallible, even in the sight of the Lord, it is when he confesses his sinfulness. Then, more than at any other time is he truthful, and when he is truthful, he attracts the Spirit of Truth, Who transforms him by the grace of repentance. This brings the believer to a deep awareness of his spiritual poverty and, in response to his repentance, the Holy Spirit grants both healing and justification.

Moreover, by repentance and confession, the Christian demonstrates his faith in God's power to save, and shows that his hope is not in man, nor in an angel, but in Christ alone Who purchased him by the Blood of His sacrifice.

Finally, repentance and confession are the cross taken up by the believer for his salvation and justification. It consists of the shame suffered in disclosing his sins to God in the presence of a minister of the Church. By doing this, he puts himself in the way of the Lord, and the Lord comes to accept his shame, however great or small, as a sacrificial offering of thanks, and in return He grants him grace which restores him. Whoever places himself in the Lord's way through voluntary shame will find that the Lord is his companion, since He said that He is the Way, the Way of both Truth and Life. Therefore, both grace and the life of the great Fellow-Traveller Himself are accorded to the believer who humbly desires the company of the Lord. In a word, by voluntarily accepting shame in confession, one not only escapes involuntary shame at the Last Judgment, but one also receives God's eternal recognition.

But grace is received in all fullness when man repents for all mankind. As soon as man's personal repentance bears fruit, God shows him the entire fallen race of Adam, and man then makes his prayer and repentance the cry of the whole earth. One often sees this in the righteous of the Old Testament. A characteristic example is that of the Three Holy Children who stood in the furnace unharmed as they repented of Israel's apostasy in Babylon, taking it upon themselves. They accepted the hellish flame of the furnace as just retribution from God for the sin of their people (Dan. 3:5–7). We also see such examples in the lives of the saints: the Holy Apostle Paul wished to be anathema for his people (cf. Rom. 9:3); Moses prayed for his people, and asked God to blot him out of His Book unless his whole people be saved (cf. Exod. 32:32). And in our own time, St. Silouan raises up to God a prayer of repentance for the whole world.[16]

NOTES

1. *Cf. On Prayer, op. cit.*, p. 133.

2. *Idem,* 'Principles of Orthodox Asceticism' in *The Orthodox Ethos,* ed. A. J. Philippou (Oxford: Holywell Press, 1964), p. 285.

3. *The Philokalia,* Vol. 1, trans. and ed. G. E. H. Palmer, Philip Sherrard, and Kallistos Ware (London & Boston: Faber and Faber, 1975), p. 123.

4. See, 'Adam's Lament' in *Saint Silouan, op. cit.,* pp. 448–456.

CHAPTER EIGHT

ON REPENTANCE

IF WE ARE TO SPEAK ABOUT REPENTANCE, we should start from the very beginning, from God's creation of man. In Paradise, Adam was held in great honour. He was angelic. He was in direct contact with God and lived in His presence. He conversed with Him face to face, and glorified Him together with the angels. He was nourished by every word that proceeded from the mouth of God. In spite of all this honour he was beguiled, as we know, by the serpent, and followed its demonic tendency, namely, to rise up against God in the desire to supplant Him. And just as the enemy had fallen from heaven like lightning, because of his arrogant desire to set his throne above that of God, so did Adam fall swiftly. The Psalmist said, 'Man that is in honour, and understandeth not, is like the beasts that perish' (Ps. 49:20).

Adam's exile from Paradise precipitated the catastrophic divide into the visible and the invisible worlds. He fell despite God's warning and his fall was of the greatest possible magnitude. However, we should think of our fall as even greater than Adam's, for we know what happened to Adam, and yet we keep on repeating the same error.

Man was created in the image and likeness of God, a 'mirror' intended to reflect all of God's virtues. These virtues are not to be understood in a moral sense, but as divine properties or energies such as wisdom, light and beauty. In Paradise, man was transparent to the grace of God; when he fell, however, the mirror of his soul was darkened and no longer reflected any of God's glorious light. Nevertheless, the gift which God had bestowed on him was so great that certain of the righteous of the Old Testament were able to catch the occasional glimpse of the Divine Light. They saw the spiritual world and bore witness to it. We remember the Prophet Isaiah who, having seen the glory of God, was called to repentance by the Lord with the words: 'My thoughts are not your thoughts, neither are your ways my ways, for as the heavens are higher than the earth, so are my ways higher than your ways and my thoughts than your thoughts' (Isa. 55:8–9). The Lord disclosed to His Prophet the extreme tension that exists between the fallen world and the 'land of the living' (Isa. 38:11; 53:8), and the great abyss which separates the two. From then on, Isaiah saw the light of this world as darkness compared to the light of the spiritual world which had been revealed to him,[1] and he mourned within himself: 'O wretched man that I am.'

Another prophet prayed in the same spirit, and his prayer is that of all the just men of the Old Testament: 'O God be merciful unto us and bless us and make Thy face to shine upon us, and make Thy way to be known on earth, and Thy salvation among the nations' (Ps. 67:1–2).

And when finally the fullness of time had come, as we read in the Scriptures (cf. Gal. 4:4), and the Lord saw that a person was working righteousness on earth and was worthy of Him, He came, bowing the heavens (cf. Ps. 144:5), and shone forth from the Virgin. 'The people which sat in darkness saw a great light; and to them which sat in the region and shadow of death light is sprung up', reads the description of the event in the Gospel of St. Matthew (Matt. 4:16). And this 'great light' began once more to speak to man, thus continuing the conversation that had been cut short in Paradise.

The Light had then been asking our forefathers, 'Adam, where art thou? Eve where art thou? What have ye done?' But neither of them answered, 'Here I am, Lord. I am hiding because I have sinned against Thee, of my own fault, and I repent. Do Thou forgive me.' Neither of them said anything of the kind; instead,

Adam cast responsibility onto Eve, and Eve onto the serpent. Adam even went as far as blaming God. 'The woman whom *Thou* gavest to be with me, she gave me of the tree, and I did eat', said Adam (Gen. 3:12), meaning, 'It is *Thy* fault.' And the Lord, Who never constrains anybody and never imposes Himself on anyone, departed. He left them to suffer the consequences of their disobedience, to toil on earth until they should 'come to themselves', as did the Prodigal Son.

Now, this 'great light' shines forth from the Virgin so as to resume the dialogue with man. But this time, God does not ask, 'Adam, where art thou?' Instead He says, 'Repent and believe the Gospel.' There are many places in the New Testament where the Lord calls us to repentance. He enlightens the world through His word, the basic message being that we should never settle for the visible order of things, because in their fallen state, they are abominable in the sight of God. Rather He teaches us that life, and life in abundance (*cf.* John 10:10), is to be gained by such conduct as is in contrast to that of the nations whose rulers wield authority and are called benefactors (*cf.* Matt. 20:25). For the Lord overturns the visible order of things and declares, 'Whoever wants to be the first, let him be last' (*cf.* Matt. 19:30; 20:26–27). He calls for our repentance: 'I am not come to call the righteous, but sinners to repentance' (Matt. 9:13), because He knows that repentance alone can heal man's nature wounded by sin. 'They that be whole need not a physician, but they that are sick,' says the Lord (Matt. 9:12). In other words, Christ comes not for those who believe themselves to be whole, who are righteous in their own eyes, but for sinners in need of healing. He comes to save them and to restore the primordial order.

And Christ's call for repentance has not gone unanswered: even before the Lord was raised from the dead, the Good Thief repented on the cross. He was evangelised; unlike Adam, he chose to abase himself, and for this reason the Lord lifted him up and granted him Paradise that very same day. Thus, the Lord shows us that whoever wants to go up and be with Him must not be afraid first to go down, for this is the true path, and He Himself has already trodden it, granting us freedom from sin and death.

Every man then, who has ever come into contact with God, both before and after Christ's incarnation – be it through hearing His word, seeing His glory, or even receiving a negative revelation in the form of an awareness of the depth of his fall – has been moved to repentance. And on the day of Pentecost, immediately after the descent of the Holy Spirit, St. Peter arose and continued to preach Christ's gospel of repentance for the forgiveness of sins.

I have found an excellent definition of repentance in St. James' Epistle. The Apostle puts it as follows: 'Lay apart all filthiness and excess of naughtiness, and receive with meekness the engrafted word, which is able to save your souls' (Jas. 1:21). From these words of the Apostle, we see that repentance implies a return to that which God gave us in the beginning: in repentance, we receive anew the quickening breath of the Lord, the very breath whereby man was fashioned in God's image and likeness. When we say that man was created in God's image and likeness, we mean that he was made in the image and likeness of His divine energies: His love, grace and wisdom. And to be able to receive that quickening breath, that engrafted immanent Word, and partake of these divine energies, we must first purify ourselves by putting away all wickedness and extirpating from our souls all that is foreign.

Whenever man comes into contact with this Word, something within him is quickened, and the primordial gift which he was given at the moment of his creation is stirred up. Man then becomes aware of his abominable state and of the truth that, bereft of God's grace, he is like a non-rational beast, and the work of repentance is sparked off in him. In other words, man can only come to true repentance if he has previously caught a glimpse of the other world; he is then in a position to see his sinful state in the light of the state he ought to be in.

It is in the 'other world' of the Divine Liturgy that we are supremely enabled to see Christ. In the Holy Eucharist we are captivated by the vision of Him Who, being rich, for our sakes became poor that through His poverty we might become rich (cf. 2 Cor. 8:9),

through Him Who laid down His life that we might live for ever
(*cf.* John 10:15; 4:9). All those things that are uttered, prayed for, and
performed in the Divine Liturgy dispose our souls to hatred of our
sinfulness, our fallen state, and we feel the need to humble ourselves
before the supreme Image of meekness and love Who is depicted
for us in the Eucharist. The Divine Liturgy should unfailingly stir
up in us the desire for repentance, the desire to amend our lives. We
also encounter Christ when our hearts receive His word. When we
read the Holy Scriptures, a little phrase often comes to life within us,
generating in us the desire for repentance. We know from the lives
of the saints that a single word can be enough to make one flee into
the desert, strengthened for the work of repentance, and finally to
become great in the sight of God. Such was the case of St. Anthony,
who heard the Gospel read during the Divine Liturgy: 'Go and sell
that thou hast, and give to the poor, and thou shalt have treasure in
heaven: and come and follow me' (Matt. 19:21), and promptly left for
the desert so as to apply it, and then became like a god among the
Desert Fathers.

True repentance is indeed a gift of God. (I recall Fr. Sophrony
saying of someone, 'That man has the gift of repentance.') This gift
is generated in us when we see Christ's meekness and love; at the
same time, we feel an ardent desire to know Him more fully. Our
yearning for our Creator occurs on the ontological level, rather
than on the psychological plane. Therefore, our vision should also
undergo an ontological shift, so that we might no longer compare
ourselves with our fellow men, but see ourselves in the light of our
Creator. Just as the incarnate Lord has a twofold nature, so must
man's nature become twofold: he must acquire the divine nature of
his Creator, not in its essential form, which is proper only to God,
but in its energetic form. And when he begins so to live ontologically,
man realises that there is no end to repentance. Fr. Sophrony used
to say that repentance is without end as long as we perceive any spot
within ourselves, because God is light, and we must become as transparent as He is. 'The more clearly I "see" God', says Fr. Sophrony,
'the more ardent does my repentance become, since I the more
clearly recognised my unworthiness in His sight.'[2]

Repentance is the turning of our whole being towards God, even as we feel a certain pain within ourselves. This pain is bitter in the beginning, because we bear the wounds of sin; but once our wounds heal up, repentance becomes sweet. One of the saints says that honey is sweet to the tongue, but if the tongue is wounded, instead of tasting sweetness, it feels pain. The same is true of repentance. When we see our poverty, we lament over it, until our lamentations are transformed into tears of love for this great God of ours.

As we said earlier on, we can never repent enough, on account of how we see ourselves in the light of the ontological kingdom of heaven; for the same reason, we can never thank God enough. Fr. Sophrony confirms that any form of self-satisfaction is an illusion which paralyses the soul. St. Paul admonishes the Corinthians, 'And what hast thou that thou didst not receive? Now if thou didst receive it, why dost thou glory, as if thou hadst not received it? Now ye are full, now ye are rich, ye have reigned as kings without us: and I would to God ye did reign' (1 Cor. 4:7–8). The Apostle reproves them for having fallen into the same illusion as our forefather Adam, who wanted to reign independently of God; and he indirectly points out the importance of spiritual poverty. In his book, *We Shall See Him as He Is,* Fr. Sophrony describes the gift of spiritual poverty as follows:

The words of Psalm 34 have proved true for me on more than one occasion – 'This poor man cried, and the Lord heard him. . . . O fear the Lord . . . for there is no want to them that fear him.' It is not at all a happy thing to see oneself as a 'poor man', to realize one's blindness. It is painful in the extreme to hear myself condemned to death for being what I am. Yet in the eyes of my Saviour I am blessed because of this very recognition that I am poor in spirit (*cf.* Matt. 5:3). This spiritual insight is connected with the 'kingdom of heaven' revealed to us. I must see Christ 'as He is' in order to confront myself with Him and thus perceive my 'deformity'. I cannot know myself unless I have His Holy Image before me. My disgust with myself was, and still remains, very positive. But my aversion begat prayer of singular desperation which plunged me into an ocean of tears. I could not imagine any possible cure for myself – there was no way of transforming my ugliness into the likeness of His beauty. And this frantic prayer, which shook me to the core, roused the compassion of the All-high God, and His Light began to shine in the darkness of my being. In profound silence it was given me to contemplate His clemency, His wisdom, His holiness.[3]

In other words, our lamentation proceeds from an awareness of our impoverishment, and takes the form of spiritual mourning. Weeping is a gift of God that unifies all the powers of the soul, and raises us to the level of the divine commandments, which enjoin us to love God with all our heart, with all our mind and with all our being. And as we try to practise His commandments, we realise that it is not we who keep them, but rather Christ Who keeps us by His commandments and restores the image of God in us.

In Paradise, Adam lived at the fullness of the commandments, but only so long as he was obedient and did not eat from the tree of the knowledge of good and evil. He possessed the gift of God, the very breath of God, and enjoyed great security, for he was established in everything good. Through disobedience, however, Adam lost everything of this blessedness. And God, in His ineffable goodness, planted another tree – not in Paradise, but in the heart of man – and it was to be kept alive by the 'rivers of water running down from the eyes of man' (Ps. 119:136). Now these rivers of tears constitute the gift of spiritual mourning, the wound of the heart, the highest form of repentance. For when man of his own free will receives this wound in his heart, he is made whole again; his being regains its integrity, and he then fulfils the commandments of God in so far as this is possible. As Fr. Sophrony emphasises, man can never reach the summit of the commandments of God, but to a certain extent, he is able to progress in them and, by so doing, he is healed.

All the Fathers greatly value spiritual mourning. We see this, for example, in the writings of St. Symeon the New Theologian, or in the letter of St. Gregory Palamas to the nun Xenia. But it is not easy to learn to weep properly. If we weep on the psychological level, we shall wither and quench all life in us; whereas if we weep spiritually, not only will we suffer no harm, but we shall be regenerated. In *We Shall See Him as He Is,* Fr. Sophrony explains the difference between spiritual and psychological mourning.[4] According to him, psychological mourning is a matter of our confining life to the visible plane. Spiritual weeping occurs when we refer every experience of ours to God, on Whom we depend for everything, for we can only lament the distance that separates us from Him.

We frequently suffer pain and hurt on the psychological level when we encounter energies that crush our heart. But we must rise above these negative experiences, and we do so by exploiting the heart-felt pain of a particular incident and convert it into spiritual energy. Fr. Sophrony often stressed that we must learn to transfer every psychological state – whether due to illness, the scorn of other people, persecution, or the incapacity of our nature – onto a spiritual level by means of a positive thought. And we do this simply by keeping our mind in the place where the Son of God is. We think on those things that are on high, as St. Paul advised the Philippians (*cf.* Phil. 4:8).

One of the Desert Fathers was asked by his young disciple how to learn to weep in prayer. He answered, 'It is a habit; a man should persevere for a long time to acquire it, with a mind always conscious of the sins he has committed and of hell. He should always be conscious of the grave, and of how his forefathers departed from this life, and where they are now.' The brother, wanting to find out more, asked again, 'Ought a monk to remember his parents who have died, and other things?' To which the Elder answered, 'Dwell on any remembrance that brings contrition to your soul. Then, if tears come, you can transfer the centre of the thoughts, which brought you to tears, to your own sins or to any other thought for repentance.'[5] (To transform psychological states into spiritual ones is the great culture of monasticism, and unless a monk learns to do that, he will never really be fulfilled in his monastic vocation, because he will encounter such states all the time. For example, a brother says a harsh word to me and wounds me. There are two ways of reacting to this energy that so crushes my heart. I can react bitterly and say, 'How ungrateful of him! I have been so kind to him for years, I pray and care for him, and look how unjustly he treats me! He is a bad man.' That is the normal psychological reaction of people in the world. But, there is another reaction. The pain is real and goes straight to the heart, but without even thinking about where this pain came from, I change the direction of my thought and I say, 'Lord, You saw my indolence and my negligence and You sent Your angel to wake me up. Have mercy

upon us.' I use the energy of the emotion and I direct my thought
to God and pray for the things I am in need of. We can always use
that bitter energy within us to pray for the forgiveness of our sins.
So I convert the psychological energy into spiritual energy, and I
enter into dialogue with God, and at the end of it I feel refreshed
and I do not even remember from where I started, or who dealt
me the blow. Thus, anything that so constrains our heart is useful
in bringing us to contrition. Fr. Sophrony encourages this disposition with the fact that Christ, whenever He was threatened with
death, did not think of it as coming from the Roman soldiers or
the Jews – He always saw it as the Cup that the Father was giving
Him. His mind was in perpetual dialogue with His Father, and He
disregarded the way in which death was threatening Him. Again,
in the Person of Christ we find our example in all the situations we
could possibly encounter.)

Someone may object: 'What do I do if this gift of the Holy Spirit
is not granted me?' Remember the words of the Lord: 'Repent and
believe the gospel' (Mark 1:15). Faith begets in us the desire to keep
the word of Christ, to test it and prove the living Truth of it; having
proved Him, we come to know Him. It is acceptable and even pleasing
to God that we should 'experiment' with Him and put Him to the
test. God Himself provokes us to do so: 'Come and see,' He says to
Sts. Andrew and John (John 1:39). 'Come and see,' says the Apostle
Philip to Nathanael who was in doubt (John 1:46); and through
them the same invitation is addressed to all of us who hesitate. In
his Epistle to the Romans, St. Paul mentions those people who have
not proved God, who have not 'experimented' with Him, and who
therefore do not come to know Him (cf. Rom. 1:28).[6] Thus, through
faith and our desire to know Him, we ask God to 'open unto us the
gates of repentance', and to grant us the gift of tears.

Spiritual mourning is reinforced by self-accusation, by blaming
oneself, and this runs directly counter to Adam's response to God
when he had fallen away from Paradise. Adam could not blame
himself, but instead attributed the responsibility for his transgression to God. He thus made himself unworthy of the gift of repentance, and God allowed him to suffer exile so that he might discover

it. We must therefore cling to the example of Christ, the New Adam, and voluntarily take the blame for everything through self-condemnation. This process joins us to the very Cross of Christ, for it was undertaken voluntarily, not for His own benefit – since the Lord was 'without blemish and without spot' (1 Pet. 1:19) and therefore had no need of repentance – but for our salvation.

Self-condemnation, then, anticipates and mitigates the judgment of God, for He is pleased in His mercy to spare us from the rightful condemnation to come. Furthermore, through self-condemnation and the consolation of spiritual weeping, we receive great hope, and we are spiritually enlarged; and although the grace of repentance sheds light on the depth of our fall, yet we do not despair, for this same grace comforts us. Whoever undertakes repentance in a sane way will therefore intensify his cry to God, Who is able to save us from the death that has threatened to destroy human life from the very beginning. According to St. Paul, it is through the fear of this death that all have sinned (cf. Heb. 2:15). The fear of death has made all people selfish and, in our egoism, we transgress in trying to survive apart from God, according to our twisted and arbitrary ways.

As we said earlier, two abysses lie before us: the depth of the mercy and love of God, shown by His Cross to which we join ourselves by voluntarily mourning over our transgressions, and the depth of the fallen state in which we find ourselves. Both lead us to intensify our cry to God, in the way of all righteous souls, and grace comes to our help and strengthens us, for it bears within itself the seed of eternal life. This seed and the consolation that accompanies it inspire us to undertake an awesome struggle with the darkness that we have discovered within ourselves, until it is all 'swallowed up by life' (2 Cor. 5:4). We stand constrained by the abyss of the love of Christ, the Cross and the grace of His Resurrection on the one hand, and the abyss of our fall on the other hand. The abyss of our fall cries to the abyss of the mercy of the love of Christ (cf. Ps. 42:7), and if we acquire this twofold vision in our life, we will never cease to be inspired day and night. In order to be confirmed in this twofold vision, we refuse to compare ourselves with anything of this earth: if we are to mourn with our whole mind and heart, we must be resolutely and exclusively fixed upon the Author and Finisher of our faith – the Lord Christ Himself (*cf* Heb. 12:2).

Just as Paradise was preserved by the commandment of God, so is our fallen nature continually restored by repentance. Repentance never ends upon earth. If it did, it would mean that our likeness to Christ-God, Who is light and in Whom there is no spot of darkness, had been perfected. The truth is that we stand in need of repentance for as long as we live and are fed by corruptible food, for our present body is subject to death. To the extent that we repent here on earth, we become like unto Him; but by His grace, we shall become infinitely more so in the life to come.

Towards the end of the Seventh Step of *The Ladder of Divine Ascent,* St. John of Sinai says that we shall not be condemned for not having performed miracles, nor for not having been great theologians or contemplatives. We shall, however, need to give an account for not having mourned sufficiently over our sins, our state of corruption, and our imperfections. For we know very well (and the prayers of our Church confirm it) that no man can live a single day upon earth without sin. This being the case, we must do our utmost to keep ourselves from sin by cultivating the new tree of the spiritual paradise which has taken root inside our bosom, and by watering it with the streams of our tears. And the One Who would be enthroned within our hearts will show Himself to be stronger than the one that rules over this world (*cf* 1 John 4:4). In other words, the presence of God must become active within us that the enemy, the possessor of this world and tormentor of our souls, be overcome. Vigilance becomes progressively easier, and we become the more able to guard our hearts from the bad thoughts that would ensnare us. Indeed, repentance is also undertaken for the sake of vigilance: when this fire of repentance and spiritual mourning begins to burn brightly in man, vigilance becomes so natural to him that no evil thought can approach; and if it dares to do so, it cannot bear the heat of this inner fire and flees. Once, on the Holy Mountain, a very good monk who is now a hermit said to me, 'We are at peace for as long as our heart is in the pain of repentance.' By this he meant that the pain of repentance is what renders the yoke of Christ easy, as it is written (*cf.* Matt. 11:29–30).

Those who were knowers of the Uncreated Light, such as Isaiah and the other prophets, as well as the saints, were inconsolable whenever they had returned to the reality of this world, and they were prepared to make any sacrifice and effort to regain the blessed state of rapture in God. This is clearly described in the life of St. Silouan. For the forty or so years after his vision of the living Christ, he was no longer able to give himself over to sleep. Christ's meek and lowly Countenance was ever before him, allowing him no rest until the very end of his life. Had he not beheld the very Countenance of the humble Saviour, as he affirmed, it would have been impossible for him to bear a single one of those endless nights of vigil and struggle; and yet he bore them in great number because he knew what he was looking for. His extraordinary inspiration did not let him find consolation in anything but God, and he describes it beautifully in his prose poem, *Adam's Lament*.

Just as prayer generates prayer, so does spiritual mourning beget more mourning, and the moment comes, says St. John of the Ladder, when man bears this mourning within himself always and in every place. Whenever he finds himself alone, he will discharge it forthwith, and his tears will fully regenerate his person. He becomes all fire in his love for God; the hatred he feels for himself redoubles his mourning, and the Lord then comes to restore him wholly with the grace that flows from His Cross.

Allow me to conclude with a passage from *Adam's Lament*, which is in fact the wondrous lamentation of St. Silouan himself:

Adam wept: 'The desert cannot pleasure me; nor the high mountains, nor meadow nor forest, nor the singing of birds. I have no pleasure in any thing. My soul sorrows with a great sorrow: I have grieved God. And were the Lord to set me down in paradise again, there, too, would I sorrow and weep – Oh, why did I grieve my beloved God?. . . . Why is it that my soul sees Him not? What hinders Him from dwelling in me? This hinders Him: Christ-like humility and love for my enemies are not in me?'. . . . Adam lost the earthly paradise and sought it weeping. But the Lord through His love on the Cross gave Adam another paradise, fairer than the old – a paradise in heaven where shines the Light of the Holy Trinity. What shall we render unto the Lord for His love to us?[7]

QUESTIONS AND ANSWERS

Question 1: You spoke earlier on the transmutation of psychological energy into spiritual contemplation, and you gave the example in the monastic brotherhood of a harsh word being spoken to someone. I wonder if you could reflect more on that and help us to understand how we, priests in the world, dealing with the multitude of people for whom we must intercede to God, can do the same in something as mundane as a meeting with the teenagers of the council, or interacting with our parishioners.

Answer 1: We should not live our psychological states on our own, we should share them with God Himself, with our Lord and Saviour Jesus Christ. The Apostle gives us just such an injunction when he says, 'If anyone is happy, let him sing. If anyone is sad, let him repent' (*cf.* Jas. 5:13). That is to say, we can transform a psychological energy into a spiritual one – not only the sad energy, but even the happy one. If we are merry, we do not live our happiness only on a human level, but we lift our minds to God and we glorify our great Benefactor by giving thanks to Him. If we are full of admiration, then again we praise the all-wise Creator. All the time we refer ourselves to Him, and this attitude is very useful especially when we receive the 'hard knocks' of life, because in such critical moments, we will find a way out and God will console us. Many times, we pray and God does not listen to us, and the temptation or difficulty remains. But one thing happens which is even more precious than being delivered from the temptation: we receive the strength to rise above it. That is an even greater miracle! All of us, eventually, will come to the threshold of death, and there is something absolutely necessary about this, because then we will have to make our choice in the most definitive way. If, when we are facing death, we remain attached to Christ and we follow Him, putting our trust in His word, this means that our faith is stronger than the death that threatens us, therefore our faith overcomes death. 'This is the victory that overcometh the world, even our faith,' says St. John the Divine (1 John 5:4). Eventually we will meet such things as will prove and test us, and we will have such a resolve that will be unchangeable for all eternity. That was the reaction of the good angels in eternity when they said, 'Let us stand well. Let us stand with fear.' They remained attached to God, while the bad angels fell. Everything was decided once and forever, because this event took place in eternity. Whereas for us, in time, everything is relative and we are only truly tested when we face death, and if at that moment our determination to follow the Lord is unshakeable, then our resolve enters eternity and we receive 'a kingdom which cannot be moved', as the Epistle to the Hebrews says (Heb. 12:28).

Question 2: Earlier, you quoted a passage from Elder Sophrony's writings, where he said that after a period of repentance he recognised God's grace being given to him and the relief that came from that. How did he recognise that, and how can we recognise that in our repentance or when we attempt to repent? And if we do not feel as if we have received that relief, is that a sign that our repentance is not sincere?

Answer 2: Yes, of course. For example, we become stronger in resisting temptations. If our stamina is strengthened against sin, that is a sign that we have found grace. If we find it easier to humble ourselves before our brother, to give the first place to the other, and be content with a humbler place for ourselves, again that is a sign that we have found grace. If we can pray with more ease, more purely and devoutly, that is again a good indication, that our state is not just psychological, but that there is grace mingled with it. There are also practical ways of testing ourselves. When St. John of the Ladder wants to give us certain criteria to check our progress, he does not say that the one who keeps vigil for three hours is on the first step of the ladder of spiritual ascent, and the one who keeps vigil for five hours is on the second step, and so forth. No, his infallible criterion is our reaction to reproof or correction. He says that if we force ourselves not to answer back when we are admonished, then we are on the first step of the ladder to perfection. If we not only keep quiet, without reacting badly, but also realise that we are wrong and we blame ourselves for our mistake, then we are on the second step. If we give thanks to God that we have been rebuked for our benefit and our correction, we are on the third step. If we pray for the one who has wronged us and consider him as our benefactor, then we are one step higher on the ladder to perfection. Moreover, he says that when someone makes a remark and we answer back, we hate our own soul. We must not have the last word. Our last word should be 'Amen' or 'May it be blessed', but we should not 'top it up' with our own remark.

Question 3: I have been struggling as I have listened to the talks with this concept of 'coming to our senses'. We live in a society that seems to be prosperous, that in a worldly sense is affluent beyond anything in history but, in fact, is utterly mad. When we hear your words, we start to see the madness all around us, and what I am struggling with is an apparent tension between the goodness of creation that still exists in spite of its fallenness and our attachment to created things. Your words about repentance and what we have to do in terms of our inner work are kind of hard 'to sell' to those who live in the world. I wonder if you can give us some words of encouragement in terms of how to present the Gospel to the world around us in a way that might help people to see that this is a realignment of priorities, so that we can change from a temporal worldview to an eternal worldview and might enter the kingdom.

Answer 3: You put the question and you gave the answer at the end as well! It is important to teach the people to set right their priorities. In the Gospel, we read that every scribe initiated into the kingdom draws out of his treasure old things and new things (*cf.* Matt. 13:52). If we are true scribes initiated into the kingdom of our Lord, then we will know our priorities and we can make all things work for the prime purpose of our life: to serve God. We may live *in* this world, but we must not be *of* this world; our mind is set on things on High. We use this world, and we are grateful to God, but our heart is not in this world, because 'our life is hid with Christ in God', as St. Paul says (Col. 3:3). We should use everything in this world with measure and discretion, without enslaving ourselves to anything, because our heart is set on things eternal and unseen, which are more real than the ones which are seen. Forgive me.

NOTES

1. *Cf. The Ascension of Isaiah* 8:21, a second-century Judaeo-Christian document which describes the journey of the Prophet through the seven heavens after his martyrdom. See *The Letters of Ammonas,* trans. Derwas J. Chitty, revised and introduced by Sebastian Brock (Fairacres, Oxford: SLG Press, Convent of the Incarnation, 1995), pp. 13–14.

2. *We Shall See Him As He Is, op. cit.,* p. 152.

3. *Ibid.,* p. 59.

4. See Ch. 4.

5. *Evergetinos,* Vol. 2, 32 (Constantinople, 1861), p. 101.

6. Note that where KJV translates 'did not like to *retain* God', the Greek text reads οὐκ ἐδοκίμασαν τὸν Θεόν, 'have not *experimented* with God'.

7. *Saint Silouan, op. cit.,* pp. 450–456.

CHAPTER NINE

ON REPENTANCE AND THE STRUGGLE
AGAINST THE PASSIONS

W E HAVE SAID THAT REPENTANCE is a general commandment that embraces all the other commandments of the Gospel. It involves the laying aside of all filthiness and malice, and the receiving in meekness of the engrafted word of God, which first brought us into being (*cf.* Jas. 1:21) and which is able to save us. We have also said that our Lord's invitation to repentance was a continuation of His dialogue with Adam in Paradise. He calls us to respond where Adam failed to do so when the Lord asked him, 'Where art thou?', 'What have you done?' He asks us to come to our senses and say, 'Lord, I have sinned, I repent, forgive me.' The Lord came in the flesh so as to resume His dialogue with man, and he exhorted men to repent and believe in His gospel. We have mentioned also that we come to repentance by the grace of God, by the very same grace which flowed from the Cross through the Resurrection of Christ, and which the Lord commanded His Apostles to preach.

Every touch of the other world brings us closer to repentance, and when the finger of God touches our heart, in that very touch we begin to discern the pattern of divine life; we observe the virtues of God and His energies. The soul is given true understanding by which it is illumined, and repentance follows naturally. We are reminded of the woman in the Gospel who lost her drachma, lit a candle, and then swept the house in order to find it (*cf.* Luke 15:8–10). A passage from the 11th Homily of St. Macarius the Great expresses this idea very beautifully:

The soul has need of a divine lamp, even of the Holy Ghost, who sets in order the darkened house. It needs the bright Sun of righteousness, which enlightens and rises upon the heart, as an instrument to win the battle. That woman who lost the piece of silver, first lighted the lamp, and then set the house in order, and thus, the house being set in order and the lamp lit, the piece of silver was found, buried in dirt and filth and earth. So now the soul cannot of itself find its own thoughts and disengage them; but when the divine lamp is lit, it lights up the darkened house, and then the soul beholds its thoughts how they lie buried in the filth and mire of sin.[1]

In other words, the true gift of repentance is felt when this lamp is lit in the soul by the action of the Holy Spirit within us, and thus does He begin to create us anew. God originally created us in His image and after His likeness and breathed into our nostrils the breath of life, and we became a spirit quickened (not a quickening spirit, for only the Lord is a quickening Spirit) and now this new breath in our heart is the beginning of a new creation, the refashioning of our person. However, the powers of the soul need to be purified and strengthened by the Holy Spirit for man to keep the grace of God's gift of repentance, and until this has been accomplished, he will be very likely to lose it. Nevertheless, once he has experienced the manner in which grace operates, he will know what to look out for. And though most of us lose grace, we must remember that the exhortations of our Lord are all eternal. For example, the Lord said, 'Take, eat, this is my body, drink ye all of it, this is my blood' (*cf.* Matt. 26:26–27), and every time we remember and repeat these words in prayer during the Divine Liturgy, we enter into their eternal reality through our invocation of the Holy Spirit. Our Lord's calling of us to repentance also belongs to eternity. And just as in the Holy Liturgy we remember those events and ask God to bring them into our lives once more, we should also remember His first call, and that first zeal and warming of the heart, and humbly ask God to renew them in us.

Saint Paul similarly stirred up the zeal of the gift of repentance in his disciples, by reminding them of their former fervour of spirit. For example, he writes to the Galatians: 'Where is then the blessedness ye spake of? For I bear you record, that, if it had been possible, ye would have plucked out your own eyes, and have given them to me' (Gal. 4:15). He admonishes them with the sole purpose of helping them to come to themselves. He does the same thing in his Epistle to the Hebrews, who were then suffering a double persecution: one by the Romans and the other by their fellow countrymen. They were in great tribulation and distress, and in order to strengthen them in the terrible furnace of their trials, he reminded them of their former zeal: 'God is not unrighteous to forget your work and labour of love, which ye have showed toward his name, in that ye have ministered to the saints, and do minister. And we desire that every one of you do show the same diligence to the full assurance of hope unto the end: That ye be not slothful, but followers of them who through faith and patience inherit the promises' (Heb. 6:10–12). St. John of the Ladder also recommends that, from time to time, the Shepherd remind his flock of their former grace, and that he stir up in them the desire to acquire it again.

Again, in the Book of Revelation, the Lord speaks of repentance through the mouth of His Apostle. At the beginning of his letter to the Bishop of Ephesus, St. John praises him for his good works, for the persecution he bore for Christ's Name, and for the orthodoxy of his teaching, but then he adds: 'Nevertheless I have somewhat against thee, because thou hast left thy first love. Remember therefore from whence thou art fallen, and repent, and do the first works; or else I will come unto thee quickly, and will remove thy candlestick out of his place, except thou repent' (Rev. 2:4–5). St. John the Divine, or rather God through him, says that we must remember our first love in order to stir up in ourselves the all-embracing gift of repentance.

One of the Egyptian saints of the fourth century, Abba Ammonas, recommends that the monk should pray day and night that God grant him the spirit of repentance. And when his prayer is answered and the spirit of repentance is granted, a circle of fire surrounds him, preventing him from falling into sin.[2]

Repentance is the means by which we cleanse the mirror of our soul, the image of God in us, and this eventually brings us to likeness to God. As we know from the Book of Genesis, man was created in the image and likeness of God. The image consists of what God placed in him, of what He breathed into him, while the likeness is man's potential which is fulfilled by living in accordance with God's commandments. And it is because of his creation in the image and likeness of God that man is able to repent at all. If we bore no such kinship to God within ourselves, it would be impossible to undertake repentance and set off on the Lord's path. But because God said so, and made it so (for His word is deed: 'He spake, and it was done', Ps. 33:9), man himself is able to work towards the showing of his likeness to God. Similarly, if the Lord had not said, 'Take eat, this is my body; drink ye all of it, this is my blood', this would never actually come to pass in our Divine Liturgy. The foundation of all being is the word of the Lord, and this is shown in the prayer of the Church in the Holy Spirit.

We must, then, be aware that God has given us to be His 'image', whereas our 'likeness' to Him is attained by the voluntary struggle of repentance. The Holy Fathers interpret the image and likeness to God in different ways; some see the image of God in man in his rational character, while others see it in his freedom. But according to St. Gregory Palamas, man's whole being is in the image and likeness of God, not just his soul, but also his body, because even the body receives the breath of God and is sanctified, as St. Silouan would often say.

We have been created for the sole purpose of showing forth the virtues of God: 'Ye are a chosen generation, a royal priesthood, a holy nation, a peculiar people; that ye should show forth the praises of Him who hath called you out of darkness into his marvellous light' (1 Pet. 2:9). And again, the Gospel says more simply that the light of God should shine through us, and then the people, seeing that, will glorify God (cf. Matt. 5:16). Unfortunately, God's image in us has been distorted almost beyond recognition, and we have yet to acquire the true likeness to Him, which we also call deification.

In order to better understand the fall of man and the need for the kind of repentance that restores in us the image of God and perfects our likeness to our Creator, let us mention, briefly, St. Gregory Palamas' classification of the divine energies. He identifies four categories of energies. The first consists of the energies of God that give substance or being to things. Inanimate creation receives only this kind of energy from God. Trees, animals and human beings possess a second type of energy, the life-giving energy of God. They possess the energy that gives substance and the energy that gives life. But man is alone in possessing the third kind of energy, the one that makes of him a reasonable creature. Finally, the fourth and highest form of energy is the deifying energy, which is given only to Christians, as living members of the Body of Christ, who are working out their salvation, their likeness to God, and who participate in His divine nature. Angels, and men who are being saved, participate in this fourth kind of energy.

Using St. Gregory Palamas' terminology, then, we can say that when Adam fell he lost the deifying energy, while the image remained, because it is irreducible and cannot be destroyed. Although God's image in man is blurred, he still posseses the third kind of energy, inasmuch as he continues to be a rational being. The purpose of repentance is to regain the fourth kind of divine energy that deifies him and makes him like unto the angels.

In other words, when man fell in Paradise through disobedience, the earth was accursed and began to produce thistles and thorns (cf. Gen. 3:18). Man, who was 'formed out of the dust of the ground' (Gen. 2:7), suffered the same fate, that is to say, his soul was subject to the thorns and thistles of the passions. Repentance therefore aims to regain man's primordial state of dispassion by means of the struggle for the divine likeness.

Because of man's fall from grace, he is weakened and unable to fulfil the commandments of God. But repentance strengthens the powers of the soul for the doing of God's will. At the outset, he receives grace enough for him to enter into the work of his re-creation. But truly charismatic repentance is a gift of the Holy Spirit, Who comes to light the lamp of the soul. But what happens to those whose lamps have not been lit by the Holy Spirit? According to St. Gregory Palamas, they must undertake voluntary spiritual mourning in faith. Again, we emphasise that spiritual mourning is not the same as the morbid introspection of merely psychological mourning, which can destroy a person. Spiritual mourning is a voluntary undertaking based on the hope that the invocation of Him Who created all things will bring a certain consolation, as it is written in the Gospel, 'Blessed are they that mourn: for they shall be comforted' (Matt. 5:4). We mourn because we have come to our senses and seen our fallen state, and we receive consolation from Him in Whose Name we mourn. We are comforted by the indescribable consolation of the Comforter, Who gives grace such as overcomes all despair, and restores us to such a firm hope that slowly, slowly, we draw near to the wondrous love of God.

In the Gospel the Lord says: '[When] they shall lay their hands on you, and persecute you, delivering you up to the synagogues, and into prisons, [and bringing you] before kings and rulers for my name's sake . . . settle it in your hearts, not to meditate before what ye shall answer: For I will give you a mouth and wisdom, which all your adversaries shall not be able to gainsay nor resist' (Luke 21:12–15). This was to be applied by the Christians who would suffer persecution, whereas we suffer very little and expect to be praised for it. In what sense, then, does this word of the Lord truly abide for ever? (cf. 1 Pet. 1:23). It does so, when we adopt the attitude of self-reproach. When we come to God and voluntarily put ourselves before His judgment-seat, accepting all responsibility for our weakness and sin, then God gives us a mouth and wisdom because our prayer of repentance has justified us before Him. He it is Who then gives us the word of the prayer, and He it is Who justifies us at the same time – and we are comforted. Furthermore, we are established for we are assimilated into the Cross and Resurrection of Christ, and into the grace and salvation which flow therefrom. However, none of this happens instantly, for it is rather a process; a stage which is referred to by the Fathers as a catharsis, a purification from the passions, from those thorns and thistles that the field of our soul started producing when we disobeyed the commandment of God (*cf.* Matt. 13:7, 22). And just as we freely gave in to temptation, so now, in the work of repentance, we return freely to God. Indeed, our undertaking of catharsis, of purification, can only be a voluntary undertaking.

The word catharsis tends to evoke a largely negative process of getting rid of something, as when we read in Colossians, 'Ye have *put off* the old man with his deeds' (Col. 3:9). In fact, the process is not limited to cleansing the house of our soul of the evil spirits that dwell therein, as the Lord said. For if we do nothing but struggle to overcome the passions, we end up sweeping our house, without ever allowing God's grace to enter in, leaving it open to hostile occupation by an even greater number of wicked spirits (*cf.* Luke 11:24–26). Instead, we must 'increase with the increase of God' (Col. 2:19) as we begin, little by little, to adorn our house with the good things of God.

The putting off of the old man with his deeds, that is the fight against the passions, is certainly a negative aspect of the process of catharsis; but we are also exhorted to undertake something positive: *Put on* the new man which is renewed in knowledge after the image of Him that created him' (Col. 3:10). We begin to understand that Christ, the new Adam, is Himself the authentic image of God in man. Christ reveals Himself as the express Image of God, because God is revealed to us in His Flesh, and we come to realise that man is *in* the image of Christ. Man is *in* the image of the Image, as the Fathers say; we are not *the* image of God, because then we would be of one essence with God, but we are *in* His image, that is to say, we are reflections of God produced by His energies.

Moreover, when God's image is cleansed in him, man overcomes all the divisive consequences of the fall, so that in him 'there is neither Greek nor Jew, circumcision nor uncircumcision, Barbarian, Scythian, bond nor free: but Christ is all, and in all' (Col. 3:11). In other words, Christ becomes our life and, as St. Paul says, we no longer live, but Christ lives in us (*cf.* Gal. 2:20). The Epistle to the Colossians speaks of Him as Head of the Body, from which 'all the joints and sinews' receive their nourishment. We must simply hold on to Christ Who is the Head of His Body, the Head of the

Church, so that His life and energy would flow into the members of His Church, that we would all gradually be filled with the divine purity of our Head. And when we receive the gift of this divine purity, we shall come to know the state of dispassion. In his Epistle to the Ephesians, the Apostle expresses his desire that we be no more like children 'carried about with every wind of doctrine', but that we, 'speaking the truth in love, may grow up into Him in all things, which is the head, even Christ', until 'we all come in the unity of the faith, and of the knowledge of the Son of God, unto a perfect man, unto the measure of the stature of the fulness of Christ' (Eph. 4:14–15, 13). This ontological growth is the result of our purification and our restoration as images of God, Who grants us the fullness and the stature, even the measure of Christ Himself.

The Holy Fathers, especially St. Gregory Palamas, speak about two crosses and two types of dispassion. The first cross is whatever we take upon ourselves in terms of ascetic effort, such as fasting, spiritual mourning, prostrations, prayer; this is the cross of *praxis*. In one of the troparia for a saint we say, 'O holy one of God, thou hast found in *praxis* a ladder of ascent to contemplation.' The cross of *praxis* is our personal effort to mortify the sinfulness of the flesh; if we do the deeds of the flesh, we shall die, says St. Paul, but if, through the spirit, we mortify the works of the body, then we shall live eternally (*cf.* Rom. 8:13). In this first cross, we try to overcome the passions, for we have not yet reached complete dispassion. When man voluntarily takes up the cross of purification from the deeds and the lusts of the flesh, a new vision will suddenly be generated within him: Christ will reveal Himself in all His Beauty, and man will surrender himself. This is exactly what St. Paul has in mind when he says that we must 'bring into captivity every thought to the obedience of Christ' (2 Cor. 10:5). In other words, we must be captivated by the beauty, the purity, the humility, and meekness of Christ, our Prototype.

We now come to the second cross, the cross of dispassion, in which the effort is no longer ours to make, for all our actions are led by the Spirit. Man becomes, as a priest in Greece once said to me, 'the horse of God', that is to say, he is captured by the vision of God, and he is then Spirit–driven, and he begins to taste of complete dispassion, which is divine.

As we undergo the purification of the first cross, there is no permanence about any state of dispassion we might experience; our spirit is still subject to many vicissitudes, because the powers of the soul are not yet cleansed or made whole. In the beginning, for example, when grace is all around us, we tend to pray a great deal and for a certain time our mind seems to us to be pure, and we live as though in another world. But we must not think that we have already reached the safe shore of dispassion. We may have achieved a certain purification of the mental powers due to unceasing prayer, but neither our desires nor our body have yet been thoroughly purified. If we believe that we have reached dispassion, we risk falling into *prelest* or 'delusion'. According to St. Symeon the New Theologian, we can hold on to grace and unceasing prayer, and proceed steadfastly on the path to God, but only when the Divine Light comes to heal our soul of her every wound.

In the life of St. Gregory of Sinai, we find that he lived for many years without an instructor in the spiritual work of the prayer of the heart. But he had great zeal, and every night he would read the whole Psalter and make countless prostrations. He prayed continually, but he did not know the art of hesychastic prayer as taught by St. Gregory Palamas, St. Paisius Velichkovsky, St. Nicodemus the Hagiorite, and the Russian *startzy* of the 19th century. He was, however, given over to every kind of asceticism and to fasting, and this is said to be worth about half as much as prayer. He excelled in virtue, but even in monasteries such people are a silent judgment on the indolent. Some of his brethren began to feel uncomfortable about him, and he finally had to leave Sinai. He went to Crete where he met some elders who were familiar with the activity of the heart and taught him the Jesus Prayer. In his biography, it is said that in spite of his ignorance about it, within just two weeks the prayer had taken root in his heart, because his heart was prepared, and all the powers of his soul had been purified by the ascetical effort he had made previously in the first cross of dispassion. We read in St. Theophan the Recluse and in other Fathers of the

Church that some people receive the gift of prayer immediately, on account of their purity of heart. Thus, what really matters is to be pure in heart; we may weep from morning until night, but the prayer will only take root in a completely purified soul. St. Gregory of Sinai acquired and mastered this great art within two weeks, because he had accomplished the work of repentance beforehand. He left Crete for the Holy Mountain, and a whole cloud of workers in prayer of the heart rose up; the Jesus Prayer spread everywhere, vivifying the entire Church.

To return to the efforts of the first cross of dispassion, prayer is not in itself sufficient to purify the soul. However, spiritual mourning does crush all the passions and heals the powers of our being. When man mourns voluntarily, invoking the grace of God, his mind and his heart become one. His whole being is unified and, being unified, it can conform to the commandments of Christ. For example, he who mourns becomes able to love, as spiritual mourning is our response to the touch of divine love. According to St. Gregory Palamas, when man finds the path of spiritual mourning, even his body is lightened through its sanctification. The commandments of Christ, which instruct us to love God with all our mind, with all our heart and with all our strength (*cf.* Matt. 22:37), are fulfilled. But how are we to love God with all our heart and with all our mind, when mind and heart are separated from each other, and the powers of the soul are all dispersed? Only in the act of spiritual mourning can the mind descend and find the heart and our whole being be unified. And this is why the Holy Fathers consider it an all-embracing virtue.

This struggle of catharsis is a very rich one. We read in Fr. Sophrony's book on St. Silouan that when St. John Kolovos (the Dwarf) was at last purified of the passions, he prayed that a last touch of these passions may return to him, because he understood that his struggle against them had been a sacrifice well-pleasing to God.[3] The words of St. Paul come to mind: 'I beseech you therefore, brethren, by the mercies of God, that ye present your bodies a living sacrifice, holy, acceptable unto God, which is your reasonable service. And be not conformed to this world: but be ye transformed by the renewing of your mind, that ye may prove what is that good, and acceptable, and perfect will of God' (Rom. 12:1–2).

Thus, the effort of catharsis is itself our reasonable worship to God; it is our daily sacrifice of repentance offered to God in prayer; it is the beginning of the royal priesthood, which is finally fulfilled in us when we reach the spiritual state that generated the prayer written on the scroll in the icon of St. Silouan: 'I pray Thee, O merciful Lord, that all the peoples of the earth may come to know Thee by Thy Holy Spirit.' That is to say, we offer to God our repentance, and when God makes it fruitful with His grace, He opens our eyes to see that the whole world is in need of the grace of the Holy Spirit, because the whole world must be saved. Whereupon, an immense pain for the whole world, such as the Lord Himself felt, takes over our heart. We see the deep pain of Christ in the words He uttered during the Last Supper: 'O righteous Father, the world hath not known Thee' (John 17:25).

In conclusion, when man finds grace in the eyes of God on account of the sacrifice he offers for his own purification, God then calls him to the higher sacrifice of offering prayer for the salvation of the whole world, in the manner of the saints. This is the perfection of God's likeness in us. This is the perfection of the royal priesthood.

NOTES

1. *Fifty Spiritual Homilies,* trans. A. J. Mason (Willits, CA: Eastern Orthodox Books, 1974), p. 81.

2. *Cf. The Letters of Ammonas, op. cit.,* p. 2.

3. *Cf. Saint Silouan, op. cit.,* pp. 67–68.

CHAPTER TEN

ON REPENTANCE
WITHIN THE BODY OF THE CHURCH

WE HAVE BEEN SPEAKING about repentance and spiritual mourning, purification from the passions and the struggle to overcome them. We said that in repentance and the struggle for purification we aspire to nothing other than the 'excavation' of the gifts which were bestowed upon us in holy baptism. All our efforts are an endeavour to retrieve the seal of the gift of the Holy Spirit, which was granted to us at that time. In holy baptism, all the gifts of the Holy Spirit were given to us. In this we are no different from even the greatest saints: we received the same gifts as they did, and no less.

At holy baptism, we become living members of the Body of Christ, because we partake of the life of the Head of the Body, which flows through it to all its members. We are united to Christ; we have 'put on Christ' (Gal. 3:26). Unfortunately, sooner or later, this grace becomes buried within us through the persistent misuse of our free will. Our effort and ascetical struggle must therefore be directed towards the cleansing, the scraping off of the layer of grime which has accumulated over the spiritual heart. As we have seen previously, this struggle for purification gradually opens up an area of spiritual activity in the heart in which each one of us may develop the gift of royal priesthood – one of the many precious gifts received by us in holy baptism.

A friend of mine once disclosed to me his discovery of this potential treasure that is the royal priesthood, a discovery which had released him from all possible thought of wanting to be ordained to the priesthood. For he had discovered the meaning of true Liturgy through repentance; his repentance had become his Liturgy. The tears he shed each night in his cell became his ardent doxology and supplication before God. I believe that when we repent, when we mourn and struggle to purify ourselves from the passions, we do indeed offer a sacrifice well-pleasing to God. This is our reasonable worship according to St. Paul (*cf.* Rom. 12:1), which conforms not to the material realities of the visible world, but proceeds through the effort of repentance to the renewal of our existence, to the regeneration of ourselves as images of Him Who is our Creator. Let us consider here the difference between repentance and spiritual mourning. Repentance is all-embracing: it includes spiritual mourning and tears. Repentance is defined by the Fathers in a general way as an irreversible turn away from sin. The works of repentance are therefore many, and spiritual mourning is just one of them, and one which is very pleasing to God. His pleasure is shown in the spiritual tears He grants us, for these are a sure sign of the action of divine love in a person. As Fr. Sophrony affirms, there is no love without tears.

When man responds to love, he realises that he is, above all, a worshipping being. The grace of God which has touched his heart enables him to perceive the Image of God, Who is the true pattern of his life, Who ignites within him the desire to live once more according to the original purpose of his creation. Grace initiates this change in him, but in order for this grace to bear fruit, he must live as a member of the worshipping Body that is the Church, the Church being the assembly of the saints through whom God speaks and in whom He is reflected. Our common membership unites us to our brethren who continuously stand before God, and this allows us to test ourselves safely, for the saints have themselves travelled the road to purification. And as members of the worshipping Body of the Church, we participate in the divine purity, which is nowhere to be found outside this Body, and we ourselves are thus purified.

Our purification does not happen mechanically; it is a matter of collaboration (συνεργία). The human will must labour together with the grace of God. In becoming a member of a club – I apologise for the analogy! – one would normally need to meet one of its secretaries. Similarly, in our desire to enter into the labour of repentance, we address ourselves to one of the 'secretaries' of the Church, that is, we seek to meet a priest who administers the sacrament of confession. We can now reveal or utter the truth about our sins, and in doing so, we put our hand to the plough which passes through the field of our soul, tilling the soil of our heart in deep furrows. As we labour, the thorns and thistles of our heart are torn up, and the field of our soul is made ready to receive the seed of grace. And if we collaborate according to the practice of the Church, this seed will bear its fruit in due time, and this fruit is nothing less than eternal salvation.

Repentance, then, is a prerequisite to our participation in all the sacraments of the Church. For the sacraments are a mystical place where the will of man meets and unites with the will of God, and our salvation lies in this collaboration. We mentioned previously that repentance is all-embracing; as such, it is the sure foundation of our life in the Church. In the sacrament of baptism, for example, by descending into the water, we promise God – and this is our covenant with Him – that we shall henceforth be dead to sin. We undergo a death at baptism, a real death. We actually die to sin, to our former way of life, to the lusts of the flesh, to the passions, to our fleshly outlook on life. We leave all this behind once and for all, and this is contained in the symbolic act of going down into the water. And because we have died a real death to sin, when we emerge from the water we receive the true life of resurrection. Indeed, we died to everything that is without value so that we might rise to everything that is precious and eternal. A covenant is made, and the whole of our Christian life consists of proving our fidelity to this covenant of holy baptism, and of living up to the honour God has bestowed on us.

The baptismal covenant is renewed in the sacrament of confession. In confession we turn to the Church, bringing with us all our filthiness, our failures, and all our shortcomings; we lay ourselves bare before the Church in all humility, and She freely grants us that which we could never have acquired of ourselves, that which we could never have attained. I say the Church gives freely: as the Body of the Saints, both in heaven and on earth, She freely transmits Her treasures of sanctity and purity to Her members. In the sacrament of confession, we receive the grace of Christ in the fellowship of His saints.

The Holy Eucharist is the crowning fulfilment of our covenant with God, the basis of which is in fact the *word* of the Lord. And the fullness of His word is surely to be found in His Priestly Prayer, in the Seventeenth Chapter of St. John's Gospel, which is now sealed in His Blood. And in the Sixth Chapter of the Gospel of St. John, the Lord speaks of the living word of His covenant and its eternal presence in the sacrament: 'As the living Father hath sent me, and I live by the Father, so he that eateth me, even he shall live by me' (John 6:57). The Apostles, however, were cleansed by the Lord even before they partook of the Last Supper. The Lord had the New Covenant in mind when He went up to Peter to wash his feet. Peter in his usual impulsiveness, said to the Lord, 'Thou shalt never wash my feet.' And the Lord answered, 'If I wash thee not, thou hast no part with me.' Peter was terrified by this prospect, and said, 'Lord, not my feet only, but also my hands and my head' (cf. John 13:8–9). In the same Gospel, we hear the Lord saying to His Apostles, 'You are clean through the word that I have spoken unto you' (John 15:3).

We have seen that we cannot truly enter into the sacraments unless we have prepared ourselves. For this reason, the Prayers before Holy Communion are full of humble repentance: we can never be worthy of the great gift of divine life. We can only entreat the Lord, asking Him to cleanse us, that we might renew our covenant with Him and participate fully in His holiness. Each time we renew our promise to God, He enables us to walk worthily of our calling to eternal life. There are times when even a desperate promise in prayer to the Lord can bring about such a renewal:

'Lord, help me through this difficulty, and from now on I will do my best', or, 'I have sinned, O Lord, before Thee, but if Thou help me . . .', and so on. Of course, man is always something of a liar (*cf.* Ps. 116:11), but a humble movement of the heart will not fail to move the Lord to grant us whatever grace we need to start again.

In passing, we note that some people have been granted abundant grace for even the merest humble thought or prayer – grace which might enable them to break away from a certain passion and never to return to it. How is it that the Lord responds so 'disproportionately' to such movements of the heart? The truth is that He is faithful in His promises, faithful in His covenant with us, and 'He cannot deny Himself' (2 Tim. 2:13). His name is 'Faithful': in the Book of Revelation He is called 'the faithful witness' (Rev. 1:5). He is faithful because He does not change (*cf.* Heb. 13:8), and His promises therefore remain forever and are repeatedly fulfilled. The word of God to our forefather Abraham testifies to the truth of this: 'And I will establish my covenant between me and thee and thy seed after thee in their generations for an everlasting covenant, to be a God unto thee, and to thy seed after thee' (Gen. 17:7). If we fail, it is because we are false, we are disloyal, and we do not honour our part in the covenant. He, however, is sure and true. Each day that we live is a grace, if only because it is given to us for repentance, whereby we enter into fullness of life, for the Lord's covenant with His people is everlasting.

CHAPTER ELEVEN

THE BUILDING UP OF THE HEART BY THE CRUCIFIXION OF THE MIND

ACCORDING TO THE APOSTLE PAUL, the wisdom of God is foolishness to the world (*cf.* 1 Cor. 1:18). The world sees only foolishness in the Cross of Christ. But anyone who has tasted of the salvation which the Cross of Christ brought into the world, knows that God's wisdom is beyond all wisdom, and that the wisdom and the power of God are able to save man.

Christ died on the Cross in obedience to His Heavenly Father, and the believer takes up his cross in obedience to the commandment of God. Man cannot be saved by avoiding the cross and death; his salvation is realised through the cross and death. Christ died on the Cross for the salvation of men, and those who desire to follow in the path of Christ, which is the way that leads to life, must willingly take up their cross in fulfilment of the divine command. They will obey God's will in the keeping His commandments and their mind will be crucified unto the birth of a new mind – the mind of Christ. To become wise, one must first become a fool, as the Apostle says (1 Cor. 3:18). One must allow one's mind to be led captive to the will of God. This is achieved in an untiring search for humble thoughts. The mind is thus preserved in blessed captivity to Jesus Christ. The study of Holy Scripture begets humility of mind, for the words themselves proceed from the humble Spirit of God. Such words must dwell richly in the believer's heart, and his mind will then become attuned to the mind of Christ.

The way of Christ and His presence in the world overturns human standards and values. For this reason, the gospel seems strange to the world. The Lord Himself says, 'I am come into this world, that they which see not might see; and that they which see might be made blind' (John 9:39). The light Christ brought into the world is such that those who think they see and are wise 'of themselves' remain forever blind, and those who do not see and understand that they are blind can really see.

The sacraments and worship of the Church perpetually initiate and instruct in the mystery of Christ's Cross and Resurrection. In baptism, the faithful die to sin and to the elements of this world, and rise to 'newness of life' (Rom. 6:4), according to the spirit of God's commandments. The Cross introduces Christians to the mystery of divine life, and in the Holy Eucharist the covenant of the Cross is renewed: whoever partakes of the life-giving Body and Blood of Christ should be dead to himself and alive to God alone. Voluntary death through faith and repentance is the right preparation for the Holy Eucharist, in which man offers his whole life to God: he receives incorruptible divine life in exchange for his transitory corruptible existence.

According to the teaching of the Fathers, there are two stages in man's crucifixion. In the first, man withdraws from the world and the passions, while in the second, which is the higher, the passions and worldly attachments flee from his heart. In the first, the believer acquires a certain degree of freedom, while in the second he is completely liberated. In the first stage, the believer overcomes the desire to exercise authority over anyone. In the second, he himself can no longer be overcome by any authority, because he is now crucified unto all: 'The world is crucified unto me, and I unto the world' (Gal. 6:14).[1]

If we are attracted by the visible outside world, we are enemies of the Cross because we are enslaved to the world. If, however, our only concern is to keep the commandments, to seek out and fulfil God's will, and to do what is pleasing to Him even if this does not suit our fallen nature, then we are 'friends' of the Cross, for we know that 'God is greater than our heart' (1 John 3:20). We know that perfect divine love has been given as a commandment. But the soul suffers because she cannot fulfil it, and so she can only pass the years of her life on this earth as one crucified.

Unless man's mind, which has been infected by the fall of Lucifer, renounces its natural understanding and accepts the foolishness of the Cross, it is not able to humble itself and take the downward journey. However, when it consents to crucifixion, then it descends into the heart, and man experiences the foolishness of the Cross as the wisdom and the power of God. Then he can stay in his heart with prayerful attention, invoking the Name of the Lord, which is why the hesychastic tradition stresses repentance as the foundation of man's spiritual ascent. His ascent is in fact a downward journey which depends on faith in the divinity of Christ and a consciousness of his sinfulness and spiritual poverty. Repentance is a fundamental gift of the Holy Spirit, and it can intensify one's sense of spiritual poverty to the extent that one lives in the world as a fool.

But the crucifixion of the mind comes mainly through obedience – a principal virtue in monasticism, and one which leads to knowledge of the will of God and to the acquisition of the mind of Christ. The dependence it occasions brings humility, which, in turn, strengthens the heart. The natural mind is crucified; the deep heart is revealed and prepares to receive the gift of the Holy Spirit. This gift is essentially the remission of sins, and having received it, the heart is free to invoke the Name of the Lord unto salvation. Thus does obedience raise man to the level of divine life and freedom.

Obedience is not a synonym for discipline. Discipline acts on the fallen man who is subject to corruption; 'that which is born of the flesh is flesh' and 'profiteth nothing' (cf. John 3:6; 6:63). Man must therefore make a leap of faith and enter into obedience. The external imposition of discipline leads to inequality, injustice and division, and is accompanied by a certain coldness of heart in both the one who imposes and the one who is subject to discipline.

Obedience, however, presupposes a relationship that is rooted in prayer. The word of God can then be born in the humble heart of one who receives the people in a fatherly way and the one who listens. In this there is no heartless cruelty. Discipline keeps the mind on outward forms and a human way of thinking, whereas obedience searches the heart and seeks to be informed by God. Discipline enables the strong to remain in power while the weak are left to perish, and this process of 'natural selection' cannot reflect the true victory of the Cross. The way of obedience, however, enables each believer, no matter how 'little' he may seem to be, to be fitly joined to the Body of Christ. He need only trust in the Cross of the Lord for his heart to possess fullness of grace.

All men, both the weak and the strong, must crucify their mind if they are to fit in harmoniously and function properly in the Body of Christ. One should not forget that Christ, the Head of the Body, wears a crown of thorns and is in this world as one who suffers. It follows that a member of the Body who avoids pain, will fall away from the Body and be separated from the Head. But if he embraces the cross of loving obedience, his heart will be circumcised and bear the Name of the Lord within itself.

The practice of keeping the mind in the heart leads to a state of spiritual virginity. Our senses can be exercised in the service of such virginity, which constitutes a crucifixion on the spiritual level, virginity being the fruit of a life which has been crucified. And the true Christian, according to the Apostle Paul, is not concerned with the outward appearance of his life, but with the keeping of the commandments (cf. 1 Cor. 7:19).

But the crucifixion of the mind by means of the commandments is an especially difficult task for man in our modern society, which breathes and cultivates a spirit of aggressive autonomy. To acknowledge the other and, what is more, to submit in obedience to the will of another, amounts to pure foolishness as far as the logic of independence is concerned. But the self-serving logic of our time is in fact a dead end both socially and in people's personal lives. The crucifixion of the mind is especially relevant today, in that it has the power to heal the egocentrism of contemporary man.

The Mind's Entry into the Heart

Man's true purpose foreordained before all worlds is attained by the keeping of the Creator's commandments, but its fulfilment presupposes the return of the mind to the heart and the restoration of its original integrity. For only then can a person love God with his whole being and his neighbour as himself, according to the twofold commandment of love. Such was the state of man in Paradise: he knew neither division nor struggle within his soul. The natural God-given power of his mind was continually turned towards the Face of God, and his delight in the glory of God knew no bounds. But now he is fallen and his mind is dispersed; he must return to his heart and rediscover his unity.

He is, however, greatly hindered by self-love, which prevents the mind from returning to and entering into the heart. Love of oneself begets vainglory in him, and this prevents him from humbling himself and believing in Christ. Vainglory darkens the heart and turns it to stone, filling it with the passionate ego, leaving room neither for God nor for his neighbour. Man becomes incapable of entering into a life-giving relationship with God, and he is deprived of the joy of fellowship with others. His mind is weighed down by its alienation from the mystical expanses of his deep heart. He is unfit for the creative work of prayer. Bereft of the consolations of prayer, he becomes unkempt and wild in his increasing estrangement from God.

Contrition and repentance are the most effective means of therapy. Contrition of the heart gathers the attention of the mind, and the compunction he feels for having betrayed and offended God, his Saviour and Benefactor, drives all evil thoughts from his mind. Through the grace of the Holy Spirit, contrition and compunction of a Christian's heart are enough to conquer all the spirits of wickedness. It was not uncommon for the saints to oppose the attack of unclean spirits with a prayer of self-condemnation rather than a word of Scripture, the former being an act of humility, and therefore the surer. Of course, Christ, being without sin, commanded the spirit of the enemy with authority and the invocation of Scripture. But man being wounded by sin is afflicted by hidden weaknesses which can be exploited by the spirit of wickedness. He will more easily chase the demonic energy away by taking refuge in the humble prayer of self-reproach, deeming himself to be deserving of every form of hardship, even the demonic.

Grace will, without fail, visit the heart for its humble disposition and broken spirit, and the mind will naturally descend into the heart and be united with it. The heart becomes a spiritual fortress, and man then receives divine strength to repel the enemies by prayer. He becomes able to chase away evil thoughts by a single invocation or even by a movement of his spirit. However, the union of the mind with the heart is, first and foremost, the fruit of repentance. The more intense one's repentance, the greater the fervour of the heart, and the firmer the foundations of the mind therein. While the pain of repentance is most effective in the mind's returning to the heart, any other pain in life can contribute, as long as it is accepted with trust in God's providence. Sickness, persecution, poverty or any other kind of suffering can be transformed into an energy which clears the entrance to the heart.

The many sufferings of men are the consequence of their continued separation from such a good God. Because of man's fall into sin, the universe is full of affliction and misfortune, and the humble Spirit of the Lord can no longer find repose therein. By His 'suffering of death' (Heb. 2:9), Christ has saved the world from its absurd and tragic never-ending chain of suffering. But Christ's sufferings, which accompanied His self-emptying from the day He assumed human nature until the time of His sacrifice at the fearful 'place of the skull' (Matt. 27:33), are qualitatively indescribable, incomprehensible and unattainable by man. Moreover, they can never be surpassed or overcome because the Lord is Love preeternal, Who, though hated and rejected by men, was appointed by God the Father to be the chief cornerstone of life indestructible and the Author of everlasting salvation.

Despite the incomparable magnitude of the Lord's sufferings, there is no element of tragedy in them.[2] Tragedy is characteristic of the suffering of fallen man, and Christ was never separated from His Father, and He fulfilled the twofold commandment of love by

His voluntary sacrifice, without ever having sinned. Nevertheless, He assumed the entire tragedy of humanity, and by His sufferings, He manifested His love 'unto the end' and so saved the world. As the path is clearly marked, so too is the pattern of life, which draws the Spirit of the glory of God to seek rest in a wondrous manner in the suffering heart of man (cf. 1 Pet. 4:14).

God 'first loved us' (1 John 4:19) and 'spared not his own Son, but delivered him up for us all' unto death (Rom. 8:32), and the believer responds to the divine summons by embracing the suffering of repentance, thus proving the measure of his love for God our Saviour and Benefactor. The man who repents plunges into a 'sea of suffering',[3] and according to the witness of St. Silouan, 'the greater the love, the greater the suffering' of the soul.[4] Yet such sufferings are not psychological. They are not the product of a nervous disorder or of some human privation or failure.[5] They are voluntary, being undertaken for the sake of the Lord's commandment (cf. Mark 1:15).

Man suffers because he has tasted of the immortal breath of the Holy Spirit, Who has kindled in his heart a yearning for God. Because he now desires Christ's infinite love, he feels that this earthly life is like a narrow prison, and his heart cries 'with groanings which cannot be uttered' (Rom. 8:26), because he cannot attain to the divine perfection of love, which has been commanded us (cf. Matt. 5:48). The believer may suffer on every level of his being,[6] but these sufferings do not destroy – they are spiritual. As a consequence of man's response to God's commandment, they are strangely linked with that incorruptible consolation which gives life to the heart and wings to the mind.

Sufferings like these confirm man's spiritual liberty, which he gains by his obedience to the divine command, as he shows his love for the great sacrifice of the Only-begotten Son of God. They also have a quality which surprises: they are accompanied by joy which conquers the passions and renders the 'law of sin' (Rom. 7:23) ineffective in man's members. And when they attain a certain measure, they persuade God to grant His prodigal servant the fire of Fatherly Love and the riches of sonship (cf. Luke 16:10–11; John 14:23). And the believer looks on in wonder as the hitherto unknown depths of his being are revealed, and he beholds himself – a person conscious of his glorious liberty.[7] Although he is unable to contain the divine gift, for 'God is greater than our heart' (1 John 3:20), his heart nevertheless opens up fully to receive 'the light of the knowledge of the glory of God in the face of Jesus Christ' (2 Cor. 4:6).

As Elder Sophrony says, the mind's descent into the heart entails suffering,[8] and yet the festival of divine love established in the heart renders 'the sufferings of this present time' (Rom. 8:18) small and of no account. Tragic falls may prove to be beneficial when seen in the perspective of the suffering of repentance, which reveal the emptiness of the soul's desolation and wound her with a longing for God. It kindles warmth in the heart and this aids the descent of the mind.

The mind's return to the heart is the second stage of its motion. The first stage of motion is its going out and its diffusion into the world, whereas the third stage is when the mind, strengthened by divine grace, refers the entire man to God.

When the mind has returned to the heart, it must remain enclosed within it and arm itself with the Name of Christ. The power of this Name offers man the possibility of mastering his whole nature and all his faculties. Thus, the grace of the hypostatic principle begins to manifest itself, and is finally perfected by the illumination of the uncreated Light.

The mind is now in the heart. God watches over it. It is immersed in the warmth of the heart, and is cleansed by the baptism of fire, which the Lord brought to earth (cf. Luke 3:16; 12:49). And when the cleansing is complete, the mind becomes as lightning, *and is ready to enter the deep heart.*

NOTES

1. *Cf. We Shall See Him As He Is, op. cit.,* p. 116.

2. *Cf.* Archimandrite Sophrony (Sakharov), Ἄσκησις καὶ Θεωρία [Asceticism and Contemplation] (Tolleshunt Knights, Essex: Patriarchal Stavropegic Monastery of St. John the Baptist, 1996), pp. 90–91 [in Greek].

3. *We Shall See Him As He Is, op. cit.,* p. 163.

4. *Saint Silouan, op. cit.,* p. 338.

5. *Op. cit.,* p. 92.

6. *Ibid.,* p. 123.

7. *Ibid.,* pp. 123, 94.

8. *Ibid.,* p. 87.

CHAPTER TWELVE

'GO IN AND YOU WILL FIND REST'

SOME TIME AGO, I heard the confession of a Russian lady, a famous writer. She was slightly confused. I said to her, 'Your mind is like a butterfly, flitting here and there, having no base; you will continually be troubled by this.' She answered, 'An old priest in Russia told me the same thing, and as he stood hearing my confession, he knocked on my head with his hand-cross, and said, "Silly woman, *go in* and you will find rest!"' When I heard this, I marvelled at the beautiful expression of the old priest, for truly, unless we find the heart, our mind will always be dispersed and we will never find rest: we will always be troubled by one thing or another, over-sensitively thinking that people do not like us, or are against us, and so on.

In answer to the question 'What is man?', the Old Testament gives various definitions. Man is defined as 'a deep heart' (Ps. 64:6). We also read that 'the heart of man seeks a spiritual and divine sensation', νοερὰ καὶ θεία αἴσθησις (Prov. 15:14 Lxx). That is to say, man, in his desire for truth, constantly seeks this 'spiritual and divine sensation', for only then can he sense the changes wrought by the right hand of God. Without this awareness of the deep heart, without this divine and spiritual sense of God within himself, man cannot be consoled, and without consolation, he cannot fulfil his task. We all need joy, peace and consolation, in order to do the work of God in a way that is pleasing to Him.

In one of the Epistles of St. Paul, we find the following passage: 'Blessed be God, even the Father of our Lord Jesus Christ, the Father of mercies, and the God of all comfort; Who comforteth us in all our tribulation, that we may be able to comfort them which are in any trouble by the comfort wherewith we ourselves are comforted of God. For as the sufferings of Christ abound in us, so our consolation also aboundeth by Christ. And if we be afflicted it is for your consolation and salvation, which is effectual in the enduring of the same sufferings which we also suffer: and if we be comforted, it is for your consolation and salvation' (2 Cor. 1:3–6). The words 'comfort' and 'consolation' appear many times in this wonderful passage, and rightly so, for without comfort and consolation, without the peace and joy that come from the grace of God, we would not be able to do our work. We would always be gossiping, criticising other people, complaining about this or that: why the lentils are not cooked enough, why the choir is not singing better, why black and not white, and so on. However, if we unceasingly attend to our heart, and try to discover that 'spiritual and divine sensation' of God within us, then there will be no time for any such thing and, what is more, all the negative aspects of our life will be eclipsed by positive spiritual activity.

In one of his texts in *The Philokalia,* St. Gregory Palamas says that those who are busy with their heart simply do not have the time to speak to anyone – not even to those who are nearest to them. Such aloofness is not, however, due to disdain or pride, rather it arises for the simple reason that they cannot forsake their precious inner work. In a way they are 'mad' about it, for they have understood that in this activity alone can man's life be fulfilled. Therefore, we must 'go in', and the rest will be added unto us.

This 'going in and finding rest' encapsulates the whole theology and tradition of hesychasm. Every Christian, whether he is a monk or not, should at least desire to draw near to this tradition. The typikon of our monastery is based on the hesychastic tradition. Fr. Sophrony gave us the two primary elements of the hesychastic tradition, namely the Divine Liturgy and the Jesus Prayer. Both of these help us greatly in realising the way of prayer in which the 'deep heart' is revealed to us.

The outward dispersion of the mind in the created, visible world and in the passions is the invention of the demons and the madness of the heathen, according to St. Gregory Palamas. St. John of the Ladder says that the true hesychast strives relentlessly to confine the immaterial mind within the material body, and we emphasise here that there is nothing evil or contemptible about the human body, which has been created to be the temple of God. But we must struggle to overcome the fleshly mind that so dominates the body, and thus make ready for the visitation of the Lord. Job asked God, 'What is man, that thou shouldest magnify him? and that thou shouldest set thy heart upon him?' (Job 7:17). In other words, 'What is man that You should make him Your goal?' And Solomon, in his consecration of the Temple to God, offered a prayer full of inspiration, which God received with the answer: 'I shall lay My name upon this Temple and My eyes will be fixed upon it' (*cf.* 1 Kgs. 8:29), and 'I shall walk among the people of Israel and I shall be their God and they shall be My people' (*cf.* 1 Kgs. 6:13). These two quotations clearly indicate the Lord's desire, wherefore we must divest ourselves of the fleshliness of the mind, that God might visit us and set His mind on our heart. But, as we know, it is no easy matter to confine the mind that it might find its place in the heart. Furthermore, it cannot do so unless it is led by the Spirit of God Himself.

When our whole being is gathered in the place where God's attention is focused, that is to say, when we stand in the presence of God with the mind in the heart, then our deep heart 'surfaces'. St. Gregory Palamas says that this process of 'gathering' oneself involves a certain amount of pain which kindles warmth in the heart. Indeed, the mind must follow a downward movement into the heart so as to be baptised in its furnace. This is the baptism of fire which the Lord promised: the mind descends into the heart to be baptised in its fire and purified as in a furnace, that it may recover its proper function. Man then regains the capacity to be in possession of his whole nature, his whole being, and to direct it towards God.

Saint Gregory Palamas says that we follow a threefold movement. The first movement occurs because of the original fall, when the mind spreads out into the visible world and becomes attached to it, thus partaking of the tree of the knowledge of good and evil. The second movement consists in our bringing the mind back from the outside world and into the heart, which is the centre of our person, as Fr. Sophrony would so often emphasise. Once the mind is bound to the heart by the grace of God – when man regains possession of his entire nature, being strengthened by that grace – then the third movement takes place: man directs his whole being towards God, his Redeemer, Who has so miraculously re-united all the powers of his soul.[1]

The purpose of all our labours as Christians is this retrieval of the heart. The heart must emerge from the thick layer of the dirt of the passions, that the mind may seek it anew. Whatever our task of obedience in the Church, whatever labours we undertake for the Church, all these should contribute to finding our heart. As for the word of God, we have only to keep in mind a few words inspired by the Holy Spirit for a spark to be lit inside us, by which we will begin to comprehend their hidden meaning, and this too will lead the mind to the heart. But the royal way to the deep heart is that of obedience. The greatest benefit we derive from obedience is the crucifixion of the mind, whereby we abandon all reliance on our fallen ways of thinking, putting all our trust in the word of God and His commandments. If we succeed in this, we shall begin to experience the wisdom and power of Him Who raises even the dead to life.

In passing, I would like to emphasise the fact that only through obedience can tradition be faithfully transmitted. Discipline is woefully impotent in this respect. Discipline and self-discipline belong to the fallen nature of man, and whatsoever is born of the flesh remains flesh and avails us nothing, whereas we seek to be born of the Spirit (cf. John 3:5) through the faith of true obedience. Discipline fails to reveal the heart, though it may be of use in the world for organising practical life. But obedience is what is needed for organising spiritual life according to the will of God, so that all our life can become a Divine Liturgy. No matter how wise and strong we may be, without obedience we will remain helpless with regard to ourselves and even more so with regard to our fellows. The strong may well prevail in their pursuit of discipline, but the weak will perish and there will be no real victory. If, however, we put our trust in obedience, humility will prevail and even those who are weak will be joined to the rest of the Body and function properly according to the divine purpose. Through obedience, each one finds his place in the Body. And whoever puts obedience first, and thereby crucifies his mind, will not fail to find his heart. It may not be among the most precious of vessels, but his heart will be filled. If not all of us can be true hesychasts, we can nevertheless be obedient and discover harmony of place in the Body that is the Church, and be firmly and fitly joined to the Head of this Body, which is Christ.

The bearing of shame, especially in confession, is yet another way of bringing the heart to the surface. How often, when our sins are confessed with a certain shame, is that shame transformed into a luminous, peaceful freedom! The mind then becomes light and free, and prayer flows beautifully and naturally; the heart experiences a different quality of tenderness which would not have been acquired even by many hours of weeping in our rooms – and this is granted to us in a mere moment of confession. Christ, Who is the Head of the Body, suffered the Cross of shame (*cf.* Heb. 12:2), and when we suffer just a little shame for His sake, He makes us akin to His Spirit, and visits us with His grace, a visitation that enlarges the heart. 'Be ye also enlarged', says St. Paul (2 Cor. 6:13).

How we need this enlargement of the heart which is the fruit of the Cross and the Resurrection of Christ! We need to be joined to the suffering Head in order to be assimilated into the mystery of His Cross and receive the fourfold enlargement, of which St. Paul writes in his Epistle to the Ephesians: the breadth and length, depth and height of the mystery of Christ (*cf.* Eph. 3:18). One of the reasons why much grace is transmitted in meetings like the one we have today is that we are the Body of Christ. Christ, being the Head, is invisibly present with us and His presence always communicates grace. The content of what we actually say is of secondary importance.

To summarise: the shame we bear in repentance and confession is one of the tributaries of the path of Christ, for it brings the heart to the surface, where we can find it. The Body of Christ was lifted up on the Cross in shame, and became the dwelling-place of the fullness of divinity, the eye of the divine brightness. Therefore, when we suffer even a little shame for His sake, He recognises us as His fellows, as kin with His Spirit, and He transmits to us His very brightness, even as we are comforted by His Spirit, Who is the supreme Comforter.

Pain is precious in the sight of Orthodox Christians; we appreciate it very much, for without it we can only be strangers to the Head of the Body Who continues in suffering for His world. Moreover, a heart that is free of pain remains cold, 'buried' as it is inside the chest. (When I went to the Holy Mountain for the first time, as a rassophore monk, I visited the Monastery of Philotheou, and there I met a radiant young monk, who said, 'We are happiest when we have pain in the heart.' Truly, pain of heart places us in the way of Christ, and the Lord refines our heart by means of pain. Fr. Sophrony used to say that we are strangers to the Holy Liturgy if we come to church without any pain of heart.) Orthodox Christians constantly strive to embrace spiritual pain both through personal ascetical endeavour and, more particularly, through the humility of a right approach to the sacrament of repentance. But in many cases, even efforts such as these do not enable us to find the deep heart. God may then allow illness to help us, or perhaps slander or persecution, as we see in the lives of the saints. Such trials enable us to find the deep heart, and then to maintain its warmth at all times, through pain and travail.

A careful reading of Fr. Sophrony's works reveals to us that he considers hesychasm – the relentless effort to 'go in and find rest' – to be the indispensable foundation for a right approach to the Divine Liturgy. He also sees it as necessary to spiritual fatherhood, for unless the spiritual father labours within his heart, he cannot be a transmitter of the regenerative grace, which procures for his children a new birth.

The people address us as 'Father', but are we really fathers? Does our word regenerate people and give them spiritual rebirth? If so, then it is right that people call us 'Father'. If not, then we do no justice to this name. Finally, hesychasm also unlocks the deeper meaning of the Scriptures. All the holy words contained in Scripture proceed from the apex of the inverted pyramid of God,[2] and if we descend towards it, to where Christ dwells, we develop a kinship with these words. To summarise: unless we crucify our mind with the evangelical precepts and make the descent into the heart, we cannot participate properly in the Holy Eucharist, we cannot help the people who come to us, and we cannot grasp the full meaning of the word of God. In short, the purpose of our life remains unfulfilled.

I would like to read you a passage from St. Gregory Palamas' *Letter to the Nun Xenia,* in which he summarises the hesychastic way. (I must admit that unless Fr. Sophrony had previously elaborated on this passage and placed us in its perspective, I would never have seen the deeper meaning of it. It often happened that Fr. Sophrony would somehow place an idea in our minds, and later, when we came across something similar, we would exclaim, 'Ah, this passage expresses what we learned and received from our father!') This passage from St. Gregory Palamas is very important to us in that it contains Fr. Sophrony's entire theory of the hypostasis, of the person. It is striking how many passages in our Elder's books reflect this one.

When... 'the day breaks and the morning star rises in our hearts' (*cf.* 2 Pet. 1:19) then 'the true man – the intellect – will go out to his true work' (*cf.* Ps. 104:23) [The true man being the one who does the true work of repentance, not on the psychological level, but rather on the ontological, as Fr. Sophrony explained to us], ascending in the light the road that leads to the eternal mountains [and being enlarged fourfold]. In this light it miraculously surveys supramundane things, being either still joined to the materiality to which it was originally linked, or else separated from it – this depending on the level that it has attained. For it does not ascend on the wings of the mind's fantasy, for the mind always wanders about as though blind, without possessing an accurate and assured understanding either of sensory things not immediately present to it or of transcendent intelligible realities. Rather it ascends in very truth, raised by the Spirit's ineffable power, and with spiritual and ineffable apperception it hears words too sacred to utter (*cf.* 2 Cor. 12:4) and sees invisible things. And it becomes entirely rapt in the miracle of it, even when it is no longer there, and it rivals the tireless angelic choir, having become truly another angel of God upon earth. Through itself it brings every created thing closer to God, for it itself now participates in all things and even in Him who transcends all, inasmuch as it has faithfully conformed itself to the divine image.[3]

This passage reminds me of Fr. Sophrony's chapter on the vision of the uncreated Light in his book *We Shall See Him as He Is*. He says that the vision of the uncreated Light causes a wondrous flower to blossom forth, whose name is *hypostasis*, or person.[4] When man is enlightened, having been enlarged fourfold, he brings the whole creation to God. Herein lies the entire theory of personhood through which Fr. Sophrony so ardently desired to help us. He describes the realisation of the divine image and likeness in man and the path leading to it, which is hesychasm. The great desire of our Elder was to enable us to descend into our deep heart and, once there, to keep our mind crucified and our heart circumcised by the folly of the Cross of Christ and the fire of heartfelt repentance, that we might receive the consolation of Christ. He was constantly trying to help us by admonishing or instructing us, consoling or teaching us, so that we would pursue our path with joy. He knew well that we are unable to accomplish our duties and wage the manifold struggles demanded of us unless we also partake of divine consolation.

Fr. Sophrony also wrote of suffering and consolation in a letter to Fr. Boris and Matushka Natalia Stark, written in 1954, on the occasion of the Feast of the Lord's Ascension. (The Starks had returned to Russia in 1952, and were enduring the bitter realities of the political situation there.)

Yes, that's it: the Ascension. The Ascent of the Mount of ascetic hardship [of Golgotha]; difficult yet crucial, and indispensable in the increase of your knowledge, and in your acquisition of that inner, moral or, rather, spiritual state, which qualifies one to converse with the heavy-laden and the sorrowful. How awkward is the word of comfort in the mouth of one who himself has no experience of affliction, who himself has never struggled unto sweat let alone striven unto blood. But where one has experience of this kind, how great the wealth and power of his word! And a priest has need of such experience more than anyone, that is, he must have knowledge of life, even of the depths of hell. Of course, he must also know the Resurrection. Otherwise nothing has any meaning at all.[5]

In one way or another, we all, and I myself first of all, are condemned by this word of Fr. Sophrony: unless pain informs our heart, we cannot transmit anything spiritual to anyone. I find his word particularly striking: the richer a man's experience, the more powerful his word; how greatly do we priests need such experience. When we come to know every aspect of life in Christ in all its depth, even the very abyss of hell, then Christ's Resurrection expands our knowledge, and our ministry can be meaningful and fruitful.

There is yet another way of finding our deep heart, and it lies in our unquestioning acceptance of correction and admonition from our elders. This is crucifixion *par excellence* of our mind and our will, and our submission releases us from schemes of our own devising, which lead us into pseudo-ascetic exploits, or some other imaginary virtue. If we have the confidence of true sons, we will gratefully accept chastisement. If, however, we turn away from our elders because of the slightest remark and assert our independence, we choose a way of folly, which is at odds with the way of the heart, and we will forever be strangers to true consolation. Moreover, without trust and fidelity to our elders we cannot be fitly joined to the Body of Christ, and our fleshly falsehood avails us nothing. If, on the other hand, we aspire to spiritual birth, inner pain and travail are absolutely necessary.

I would also emphasise the great importance of the traditions instituted in and by the Holy Spirit. We must honour them with our lives and avoid putting our fallen reasoning above them. Indifference to the Holy Spirit is a common cause of stagnation in spiritual life and it leads to an inability to embrace tradition. But let us not remain stuck in our fallen mind. Our Church encourages us to establish a solid base for ourselves so that our mind can be right within us; instead, we often 'provoke one another, bite one another and in the end even consume one another', as St. Paul says (*cf.* Gal. 5:15). St. John of the Ladder, in describing monastic spiritual perfection, classifies the monk according to the way he responds to insults and remarks, and to chastening by his elders. Let us note well that his criterion has nothing to do with correct behaviour, prayer rules, or prostrations. Of course, these things may be good, but there is nothing like a word of correction to put our intentions to the test. If we are angered by even a small reproach, then it is obvious that our efforts are in vain. We often lose sight of the importance of trust. Fr. Sophrony used to point out that spiritual fathers rarely test anyone because they know well their own measure, and are fearful of being too daring. However, a small number of fathers have the gift of discernment, and are able safely to lead their disciples to the very threshold of death. Needless to say, they do not aim for the death of their disciples, they rather yearn for them to mortify their old habits and their old selves; they yearn for their regeneration, and to make them sons of God. Now that we know of the great benefits of enduring a 'hard saying', let us be attentive to seize the first such saying that is presented to us; let us crown it with silence, rather than drowning it with ten more words of our own!

Truly, I cannot labour the point enough: if the institution of the Church is not given the respect and love that She is due, then Her Tradition, which has been so beautifully recapitulated in St. Silouan and Fr. Sophrony (who did his utmost to transmit it to us), will simply remain inaccessible. We will not be able to assimilate it, let alone to pass it on in our turn. We will just be a bunch of nice people, who – God forbid! – allowed the Tradition of true life to die along with them. The path has been trodden and the rules have been laid down: we have nothing to invent. Forgive my daring to say so, but nothing is too difficult for anyone who has the desire to follow this path in mindfulness of the exhortations of our Tradition, and embracing those things which unfailingly place us in the way of Christ, which is also the way of our Fathers in God.

QUESTIONS AND ANSWERS

Question 1: You discussed things that cause trouble in our journey to find the heart: we have weakness in our body and in the mind. You also mentioned that one of the things that causes difficulty is our society that we live in, based on pride. In another talk, you mentioned that it is very helpful to withdraw from that understanding of life in order to find our heart. Can you give us some insights on the phenomenon of the 'fool for Christ' that would help us understand how to deal with the world around us, which we are immersed in, and how that would help us in our journey to find our heart?

Answer 1: To be a fool for Christ's sake is a very special gift in the Church. Those who have undertaken that kind of life were people who had great blessings and, wanting to hide them, they found ways of provoking the contempt of the people around them in order to keep the humility necessary to preserve the great gifts that they had received. Fr. Sophrony told me once that those people who became fools for Christ also had something in their nature convenient for that kind of life. It is not for everybody. He told us that once on the Holy Mountain somebody went to a great Elder to ask his blessing to become a fool for Christ, and the Elder said to him, 'No! Now it is not the time for that. Nowadays even by keeping the faith in the world we are fools for Christ's sake!' That reminds me of the saying of a Father from the fourth century. When asked, 'What have we done in our life?' he answered, 'We have done the half of what our Fathers did.' When asked, 'What will the ones who come after us do?' he replied, 'They will do the half of what we are doing now.' And to the question 'What will the Christians of the last times do?' he replied, 'They will not be able to do any spiritual exploits, but those who keep the faith will be glorified in heaven more than our Fathers who raised the dead.'[5] In general, I think the way of the Gospel is foolishness to the world. As St. Paul says, if you want to become wise, you first have to become a fool (*cf.* 1 Cor. 3:18).

Question 2: What struck me when you were talking about the life of St. Silouan was the fact that after he had the vision of Christ he felt almost sad with longing for that. I think that even if we do not relate completely to that, nevertheless, we know from our lives at some definite points, whether it is in the Divine Liturgy, or while reading the Bible, that God touches our heart in a very concrete way, and we feel His presence. Maybe we do not have the vision of Him, but we feel His presence and it is very comforting, but those moments are rare. Is it wrong to long for that? Do you question why God does not touch our hearts more often? Is it something that we do right when God touches our heart and something we do not do right when He does not?

Answer 2: Those moments are the great moments of God's visitation of us. In the Epistle to the Hebrews St. Paul says to his disciples that they should remember those days when they were full of grace, showed much zeal and were ready to suffer (*cf.* Heb. 10:32). Those moments bring a tremendous strength to our life, because we know that we always have the same possibility, that through God's grace we can have contact with Him, because He is the living God, He is risen from the dead, He lives and reigns for ever. We have the possibility to have contact with Him, to experience His living presence. The memory of those things should stir up the desire for God and even help us to overcome temptations. We must always seek God's help, and knock at the door and ask, but it is up to God's discretion when to give grace to us. When He does not give us grace, it is not because He is mean, but because He foresees that we are not able to keep it, and He does not want to make our lives even more difficult. He waits until we become more mature in spirit, so as to bestow His gifts on us at a time when we may be able to keep them. From the lives of the saints we know that our existence becomes a torment when we know the great mercy of God and then lose it, because nothing else can give us pleasure, as we read in St. Silouan's *Adam's Lament.*

Question 3: Earlier you drew a dichotomy between the term self-discipline and obedience. St. Paul seems to talk about what I would call self-discipline when he says, 'I buffet my body so that I won't be disqualified.' I suspect there is some semantic difference. Would you elaborate on the difference between self-discipline and obedience, and how discipline is necessary for obedience?

Answer 3: I was talking about discipline as we know it in the world. It is through discipline that the world is organised, and this discipline tends to be imposed. Obedience is a free undertaking because of our faith and trust in God, and because we want to imitate the example that He showed us. Self-discipline is, of course, valuable. We all try to do something day by day, and that is not to be despised, but it is not as beneficial and great as obedience. Self-discipline is a voluntary undertaking and if it is done for God, it has great value, but obedience is a total sacrifice because what is most precious to man is his free will, and he lays it at the feet of Christ, voluntarily. That is why it has such power.

Question 4: Father, I do not want to disappoint you with this question, because it is likely to be very elementary, and probably something that most people already understand. My question is linked with the things that you said about finding the heart and entering into it. Oftentimes when I think about this and I seek it praying, or at Divine Liturgy, it is as though I am looking for something that when I find it, I am able to carry it around in my hands, metaphorically speaking. But you said that when you enter into your heart, the heart expands and then is located everywhere within you. I am wondering if I understand correctly that the heart is that truth that you find about yourself and God through repentance and confession, Divine Liturgy and prayer. Is it in a sense more a way of living, a mode of existence rather than a lifetime point of contact, if I am making any sense?

Answer 4: When we find our heart, the first thing that we know is that we belong entirely to Christ, that we are His and we have a certain strength, and each invocation of His Name is in the power of His Spirit. It is not an easy thing to describe. We always pray, but each time we do it, it is different. Sometimes we pray and it is very painful and difficult, while at other times we cannot abandon prayer, but prayer carries us. Occasionally, we make an effort and God comes to our help. It always changes. However, when we really find the deep heart, it is as if we have thrown out an anchor, not into the sea, but into heaven, and this anchor draws our whole being to Christ, and we know that we belong to Him.

Question 5: How are we who are not in the monastic life to find the sources for our obedience in the world, so that we know that we are offering true and humble obedience to God and His will?

Answer 5: Obedience in a specific way is only for monasteries, because there everything is organised around the Divine Liturgy, everything functions with this purpose. Nevertheless, obedience

is important for every Christian, and for the priest. First of all, he
has his obedience to his bishop, and that protects him enormously.
If the relationship of the priest with his bishop is straight and as
it should be, then this is a great strength for the priest. Surely
the priest has a confessor and, of course, when he asks for a word
from him, he will consider it seriously. When we have this spirit
of obedience we can be helped easily; we do not need wonder-
working priests in order to be obedient. We need someone who is
willing to listen to us and help us and who has a valid *epitrachelion*.
For those of you who are married, even obedience to your wives is
beneficial. You must listen to your wives, because sometimes they
can be very intuitive and see things better than you do. I knew a
priest who, when he was in great temptation and had no spiritual
father near him to confess to, went and confessed his problem to
his wife. Fortunately, his wife was a spiritual person as well, and
she listened with discretion and gave him the right advice. He
followed her advice and was saved. He would have perished if he
had not done that.

A Brief Comment: In his book *Orthodox Psychotherapy,*
Metropolitain Hierotheos Vlachos includes a prayer of St. Symeon
the New Theologian, in which he asks God to help him to find a
holy elder: 'O Lord, who desirest not the death of a sinner but that
he should turn and live, Thou who didst come down to earth in
order to restore life to those lying dead through sin, and in order to
make them worthy of seeing Thee, the true Light, as far as that is
possible to man, send me a man who knows Thee, so that in serving
him, and in subjecting myself to him with all my strength as to
Thee, and in doing Thy will in his, I may please Thee, the only true
God, so that even I, a sinner, may be worthy of Thy kingdom.'[6]

Response: The author of this book is a very good friend of mine.
I have known him since 1972, and we have been very closely linked.
He is also an experienced monk and now a bishop. And, you know,
his spiritual father was his own bishop, and though his bishop
perhaps did not know as much as he did about hesychastic prayer,
nevertheless he had the discernment to understand what was
going on in him, and to give him the freedom to pursue that kind

of prayer life. He protected and shielded him, and he developed and became a man of prayer and a true teacher of the Church.

NOTES

1. *Cf.* St. Gregory Palamas, 'The Hesychast method of prayer, and the transformation of the body', in *The Triads* (New York, Ramsey, Toronto: Paulist Press, 1983), trans. N. Gendle, p. 44.

2. For Archimandrite Sophrony's theory of the 'inverted pyramid', see *Saint Silouan, op. cit.,* pp. 237–239.

3. St. Gregory Palamas, 'To the Most Reverend Nun Xenia', in *The Philokalia,* Vol. 4 (London: Faber & Faber, 1995), pp. 316–317.

4. *Cf. We Shall See Him As He Is, op. cit.,* p. 186.

5. Archimandrite Sophrony (Sakharov), Письма Близким Людям [Letters to Close Friends] (Publishing House, "Отчий Дом", 1997), pp. 45–47 [in Russian].

5. *Cf.* Abba Ischyrion in *The Sayings of the Desert Fathers: The Alphabetical Collection,* trans. Benedicta Ward (Kalamazoo, MI: Cistercian Publications, 1975), p. 111.

6. 'In Quest of a Spiritual Healer' in *Orthodox Psychotherapy,* trans. Esther Williams (Levadia, Greece: Birth of the Theotokos Monastery, 1994), p. 356.

CHAPTER THIRTEEN

THE DEEP HEART,
NEW ENERGIES AND TRUE HUMILITY

TODAY'S SUBJECT IS SO DEEP and great that I cannot rely on my insufficient prayer, or preparation, but I rely more on you who are better than I, since we are all one Body in Christ. The Holy Spirit was given to the Church as one Body on the day of Pentecost, when all the Apostles were gathered together. There is in Greek the term *synchorisis*, which means to find the *choros*, the 'place' where we are all contained, namely, the Spirit of God in Whom we are all embraced. *Synchorisis* also means to bear everyone in our heart, making room in our heart for everyone, and if anyone is excluded, then we are not truly in that *choros*, which is the kingdom of God. Historically speaking, the Holy Spirit came upon the assembly of the disciples, who were gathered together on that first day of Pentecost, and the climax of this great feast of God will take place in heaven where one day we shall all be united together.

We read in the Book of Revelation that the saints are waiting under the altar of God with a mixture of expectation and, perhaps, uncharacteristic complaint. 'I saw under the altar the souls of them that were slain for the word of God, and for the testimony which they held: And they cried with a loud voice, saying, How long, O Lord, holy and true, dost thou not judge and avenge our blood on them that dwell on the earth?' (Rev. 6:9–10). But, in our favour, God foresaw a better end than this, as we can see in the Epistle to the Hebrews: 'And these all [who have been saved, from the beginning till the end of time], having obtained a good report through faith, received not the promise. God having provided some better thing for us, that they without us should not be made perfect' (Heb. 11:39–40). The Apostle lets us understand that although the saints wrought righteousness and obtained the victory and the martyrs shed their blood, they have not yet been made perfect. It is as if they had received breakfast but are not yet enjoying dinner in the kingdom. God has indeed provided better things because He wants all peoples to taste of that great feast of divine love after the general resurrection. And it was for this very reason that the Spirit of God was given to the Body as a whole. 'Thou hast perfected a body', says Scripture (Heb. 10:5); Christ has indeed perfected the Body of His Church throughout history, and in His kingdom He will give full glory to the whole Body. We may be insignificant members of this Body, but He will still include us in the great feast of divine love. Therefore we cannot be jealous of one another because the Head imparts all that He has to each of the members of His Body, from the greatest to the least. Fr. Sophrony used to speak of the godly contest that takes place in heaven: the saints are in such a blissful state of humility that they rejoice upon seeing their fellows in greater glory than they are themselves.[1]

As it is, the saints still await the fullness of grace. They are clothed in white garments, and in a way they are feasting already, but the fullness of the feast will come only when they have been joined by the whole number of the elect. Those still living will be transformed together with those who are already risen from the dead, and all will thus be made perfect together.

Such, according to St. John Chrysostom, is the economy of God. In ordering things this way, He does not wrong the saints, but He rather honours us. We recognise this way of the Lord in the parable of the householder who went out early in the morning to hire labourers for his vineyard, and at the end of the day gave the same wages to those who came at the last hour as to those who had come at the first hour (cf. Matt. 20:1–15). Just as the lord of the vineyard was in no way unjust in being generous to the last to come, neither does God wrong those who are already in the kingdom. He simply wants to honour us for whom the saints are waiting. The saints, who have been crowned and have the same spirit of philanthropy as their Master, wait to rejoice with us in the common glory of the whole Body. In other words, the end of all good things will be this perfection which we all await in patience. (These thoughts bring me consolation as I speak to you who are better than I – I do not rely on my preparation, nor on my own words, but on the prayers of this Body.)

God has given a great honour to the body of man in that He made it the temple of His Spirit, and the body most interior to this body, as St. Gregory Palamas calls the heart,[2] is the place where His kingdom is manifested. Therefore, it is no small thing if we establish our mind in the presence of God, in the place before the footstool of the great King. We would do well, then, to direct our efforts towards going inwards and establishing ourselves in the deep heart.

Great potential energy is hidden in our deep heart. If, at prayer, we are weighed down by the thought, 'Oh, I am exhausted, I can't go on any longer', and we then turn to the Lord with pain in the heart and say, 'Lord, You see, I am tired. You deserve better things which I cannot offer. Forgive me.' And this little thought of humility on our part immediately releases a new energy, and prayer can continue. And if again, overcome by tiredness, we say, 'Lord, I had desired not to interrupt my conversation with You, but You see I have no strength left', this humbling of ourselves provides a further burst of energy to refresh and strengthen our being. Therefore, in order to tap those energies that enable us to carry on with God's work, it is indispensable that we find the deep heart.

Fashioned in the image and after the likeness of God, man has been endowed with great potential by his Creator. If we consider that everything came into being through the word of God, and that His word has the power to regenerate the whole creation, what shall we say of the word of man? The Gospel says that every word uttered by man will live until the Last Judgment, when he will meet with it again. By assuming man's nature God also endowed man's word with power, making of it a means of transmitting His revelation. Moreover, the greatness of the human word lies in its eternal quality, for it is through Christ's word, the Word of God made man, that God performed the miracle of universal regeneration in Christ. Fr. Sophrony says in his book *On Prayer* that although Christ uttered human words, in those human words He revealed divine mysteries.

One of the mysteries revealed by the word of Christ is that of the kinship between the heart of man and the presence of God. And therefore a sure path to discovering and establishing ourselves in the deep heart lies in meditation on the word of God and the invocation of the Name of Christ. It is said, by the witness of the Holy Spirit which was received at Pentecost, that 'there is none other name under heaven given among men, whereby we must be saved' (Acts 4:12). Moreover, we read in the second Epistle to the Corinthians that the word of God must dwell richly in our heart and bring all our thoughts captive to the obedience of Christ (*cf.* 2 Cor 10:5). Both meditation on Christ's word and invocation of His Name are perfected when we partake of the Holy Body and Blood of Christ. It is said in the Gospel of St. John that unless we eat the Flesh and drink the Blood of the Son of God, we cannot have life in us (*cf.* John 6:53).

To summarise, the keys that open the door to the deep heart are: meditating on the teaching of the Gospel, calling upon the Name of the Lord, and partaking of the sacrament of Holy Communion. All three of these keys release the energy contained in the deep heart. We are invested with this energy at baptism, but we bury it through our sinful living, our ignorance and negligence. Let us uncover the divine treasure that lies concealed within us by fixing in our mind some inspiring words of God, and trying to deepen our fervour for Holy Communion in the Body and Blood of Christ. And let us persevere in calling upon the Name of our Lord Jesus Christ, which has been given by revelation, and which is inseparable from the Person of Christ, and therefore able to transmit His saving energy to us.

In his book *On Prayer*, Fr. Sophrony also points out that when we gather all our being and install our mind in the deep heart, the entrances of the soul are protected against the temptations of the evil one, and only then do we stop falling into sin. This is also the moment when we become truly humble. The saints have given us many definitions of humility, but personally, I like that of St. Maximus the Confessor. According to him, humility is to know that we have our being 'on loan' from God,[3] an acknowledgement that fills our heart with gratitude. Saint Maximus also emphasises the significance of gratitude, saying that gratitude is equal to humility.

There exist different degrees of humility. According to Fr. Sophrony, however, man acquires true spiritual humility and finds his heart when he comes to realise that he is unworthy of such a God as Christ. Humility then enables him to receive and accept the revealed truth that Christ has given us. And in accepting it, he is given grace, and this grace functions as a tour-guide in our heart, allowing us to see all its uncleanness and filthiness, and giving us the courage to say, 'Yes, Lord, I am a filthy rag, I am dust and earth. I am a worm and not a man (cf. Ps. 22:6). I am the chief of all sinners', to borrow from the words of prayer of the Prophets and the Apostles. True humility involves sincerely standing before the truth revealed in Christ and confessing the uncleanness and filthiness which we bear hidden within us without realising it. The grace of God then sheds light upon our darkened soul, and in His light we see our own light. 'In Thy light shall we see light', as we sing in the Doxology (Ps. 36:9). Only when God illumines us by His grace are we able to see the true light of our own existence.

For Fr. Sophrony there is no greater miracle in the world than this moment when the Uncreated unites with the created. He pursued this very miracle all his life both for himself and for the people who came to seek his help. He never sought to be a wonder-worker, and attached no significance to the miracles that occurred through his prayers. But when the greatest miracle in existence took place, that is, the union of the created with the Uncreated, our Elder would rejoice, even if the person were dying physically.

This miracle is analogous to the Big Bang of the astronomers, and to the words in Genesis: 'Let there be light and there was light.' When it takes place in the heart of man, it reveals the 'true man'.

We recall the words of St. Gregory Palamas in his *Letter to the Nun Xenia,* based on St. Peter and the Psalms: 'When the day will dawn and the morning star rises in your heart, the true man will go out for his true work.'[4] St. Gregory Palamas describes in beautiful poetic and theological language this spiritual event that occurs when the rays of uncreated Light penetrate our being, and the 'deep heart' opens, and man begins his 'ontological work'.

Again, I would like to refer to and make some comments on a few passages from Fr. Sophrony's writings, which parallel this quotation from St. Gregory Palamas. The first text is from Fr. Sophrony's book *On Prayer,* and it begins with this exhortation: 'Keep your mind firmly fixed on God.' How else can we keep our mind fixed on God but through the invocation of the Name of Jesus Christ? For His Name is inseparable from His Person and by fixing our mind on the Name of God, we live in the presence of His Person. For this reason, St. Theophan the Recluse advises the following in his letters, 'As soon as you rise up in the morning, establish your mind in the heart, in the presence of God, and wind up your clock to run all day!' It is important to make a good beginning by setting our mind in the heart, and dwelling in the presence of God through the invocation of the Name. In one of his meetings with us, towards the end of his life, Fr. Sophrony urged us: 'Do not come to the service without warming your hearts with prayer. Before coming to the service, pray for at least ten minutes. Come ready to stand in the presence of God, for the invocation of the Name! Those of you who have the strength, do it for one or two hours, but you should do it for at least ten minutes. Do not neglect it, otherwise you will dry up!'

This continual invocation of the Name is a commandment that we have received from the Lord. In the parable of the judge who did not fear God, the widow persisted in troubling him until he did justice to her (*cf.* Luke 18:2–7). If this judge, who was unjust, yielded in front of her perseverance, how much more will our Lord, Who is a God of love and justice, hearken unto one who, day and night, cries to Him in prayer? Therefore, it is a good thing to increase our presumption, our daring towards God, in order to pray continuously, because God likes it when we force Him: 'Until now the kingdom of heaven suffereth violence, and the violent take it by force,' says the Gospel (Matt. 11:12). He likes it in that He recognises our potential to be equal to Him. Prayer of the heart is a divine commandment, and by fulfilling it, we put ourselves in the way of Christ and He becomes our companion.

If we read Fr. Sophrony's writings carefully, we shall understand that he considers the Jesus Prayer to be a precondition both for proper participation in the Divine Liturgy and for carrying out the ministry of reconciliation, or spiritual paternity. Unless we prepare our heart by continually calling upon the Name of the Lord, the heart cannot 'snatch' the word of God and be revived by it. This applies even more to the ministry of confession.

But let us take a look at Fr. Sophrony's own words: 'Keep your mind firmly fixed on God [or 'Wait upon the Lord', as the Psalmist would say (*cf.* Ps. 37:9; 123:2)] and the moment will come when the Immortal Spirit touches the heart. Oh, this touch of the Holy of Holies! [This is the Big Bang!] There is naught on earth to compare with it – it sweeps the spirit into the realm of uncreated Being. It pierces the heart with a love unlike that which is generally understood by the world. Its light streams down on all creation, on the whole human world in its millenary manifestation. Though this love is sensed by the physical heart, by its nature it is spiritual, metaphysical.'[5] In other words, when the great miracle of his existence occurs, and man is enlarged by the love of God, then his heart embraces all the ages and the whole creation.

This is a beautiful text, and we do not have to be great ascetics to see that happening in us; all we have to do is to keep hold of the gift that Christ has entrusted to us. St. Paul says, 'I laboured more abundantly than they all: yet not I, but the grace of God which was with me' (1 Cor. 15:10). If we are humble and serious about the gifts of God, then His grace and consolation do the work of God in us. We need the consolation of God and we must treasure it, because this grace will make the invocation of the Name of God easier and build up in us the inner strength we need. This inner strength must accumulate so as to fortify all the faculties of the soul which enable us to bear that great moment, that Big Bang, when we shall be born into the everlasting kingdom.

Father Sophrony also writes: 'It is vital to continue in prayer for as long as we can, so that His invincible strength may penetrate and enable us to resist every destructive influence. With the increase of this strength in us comes the joy of hope in the final victory. [In other words, grace generates grace: 'God grants prayer to him that prays and He blesses the years of the righteous,' says the Old Testament (1 Kgs. 2:9 Lxx).] Prayer assuredly revives in us the divine breath which God breathed into Adam's nostrils and by virtue of which Adam became a living soul. [Therefore, perseverance in the single thought that is the Jesus Prayer restores the primordial breath of God in us.] Our spirit, regenerated by prayer, begins to marvel at the sublime mystery of being.'[6]

When this great miracle occurs, everything in us functions in such a way as to bring us to a greater fullness of the love of God. 'We know that all things work together for good to them that love God,' says St. Paul (Rom. 8:28). But this happens only when the powers of the soul receive the strength of the breath of God to function properly. Then all that we see, hear and touch will provoke in us humility, contrition, love and gratitude towards God. You may hear, for example, a pop-song in a bus, and yet not be disturbed by it, but on the contrary, find something positive in it that keeps your being immersed in the love of God. Thus, when we are born again from on High, the divine grace in us finds a way of transforming even the most trivial and negative things into something positive and edifying.

Let us return to Fr. Sophrony's description of this spiritual event. 'The mind is filled with wonder. "Being, how is it possible?" And we echo the Psalmist's praise of the wondrous works of the Lord.'[7] Indeed, we remember the words of the Psalm: 'The heavens declare the glory of God; and the firmament showeth his handiwork' (Ps. 19:1). We acknowledge that there is a great liturgy of the whole universe, celebrating the love of the Creator, and we enter into that cosmic doxology, as did the nuns at Aegina after the prayer of St. Nektarios. 'We apprehend', says Fr. Sophrony, 'the meaning of Christ's words, "I am come that [men] might have life, and that they might have it more abundantly." "More abundantly" – this is indeed so.'[8]

There is another passage in Fr. Sophrony's book *On Prayer,* similar to the one we have just mentioned. 'How radically everything alters when the heart suddenly opens to accept Christ's summons! Every moment becomes precious, full of profound meaning. Suffering and joy wondrously merge with new ascetic striving. The ladder to the skies is set up before our eyes. "Thy name shall be called . . . Israel; for hast thou power with God and with man, and hast prevailed" (*cf.* Gen. 32:28–29).'[9] According to the Jewish interpreters of the law, 'Israel' is a specific term designating 'a mind that beholds God'. We, too, must acquire this mind that beholds God, because if we do so, things become much easier, and the commandments of God no longer seem like a huge mountain, too difficult for us to climb.

Due to our fallen state, we rebel in affliction, we mourn and we complain; and in joy, instead of enlarging our heart, we enlarge our mouth, thus losing all the strength that this joy contains. In order to be perfect hesychasts, we must be like the Mother of God; we must learn how to enlarge our heart, and then keep and ponder everything in it, and be silent. In the Akathist Hymn, the Mother of God is called 'a vessel sealed by the Holy Spirit', because she kept everything in her heart (*cf.* Luke 2:19). She spoke only once, when she met Elisabeth, who then confirmed the truth of the great event that was to happen – the birth of Christ. And at that moment, the prophetical gaze of the Mother of God included even the end of time when she said: 'Behold, from henceforth all generations shall call me blessed' (Luke 1:48). From then on, she lived in total surrender to Him Whom she had conceived through the Holy Spirit, never uttering a word even when her life was in danger. Ever since then, we do indeed call her blessed, and in this we fulfil her prophecy.

Many times Fr. Sophrony spoke to us about the dangers the Mother of God faced, and how she allowed nothing of the fragrance of the Holy Spirit invested in her heart to escape, whether she was in great joy or in tremendous affliction. It was unheard of for a virgin to conceive. Therefore, even though Joseph was a just man (in the language of the Scriptures this meant that he was above the laws of the flesh and led by the Holy Spirit), he was confused and suspicious. Nevertheless, the evident holiness of her person would not permit him to make of her a public example: under Jewish law she would normally have been stoned. His solution was to quietly abandon her. But even as the danger of death increased day by day, her perfect faith, hope and love in Him Whom she had conceived were stronger than any danger. Her heart was sealed. And when later she saw the angels of God going up and down above the cave at Bethlehem, and the reverent magi uttering their wondrous words, and the shepherds bringing witness to the miracle, she silently kept all things in her heart, as the Gospel says (cf. Luke 2:51). Likewise, she uttered nothing when St. Simeon the God-receiver took Christ in His arms and called Him 'a light to lighten the Gentiles, and the glory of thy people Israel' (Luke 2:32). These were conventional terms used to designate the divine Messiah, and Simeon the Righteous was in fact proclaiming Him to the Jews as the Messiah, Emmanuel, the Saviour of the world for Whom all were waiting. Addressing the Mother of God, he then said that a sword would pierce her soul (cf. Luke 2:35), prophetically alluding to the moment of Christ's crucifixion, when she would see the Life of all hanging upon the Cross. Again, at that moment, although her pain was greater than anybody else's pain could ever be, she never once opened her mouth, whereas those present smote their breast and departed (cf. Luke 23:48). The Mother of God stood by the Cross in a godlike manner, bearing a pain which was deeper than all human pain because her love for her Son and her God was deeper than anyone else's. She was all perfect, and neither in joy nor in affliction would she open her mouth, and in this she fulfilled the words of the Wisdom of Sirach, 'I brooded on nine thoughts in my heart and the tenth I uttered with my mouth' (cf. Ecclus. 25:7). For if we open our mouth in joy, we risk falling into vainglory, we risk provoking others and losing grace; if we open our mouth in suffering, we risk falling into rebellion, into bitterness or complaint.

With this in mind, we might add that the ministry of those appointed by the Church to teach the word of God is a perilous one. St. James the Apostle warns us, 'My brethren, be not many masters, knowing that we shall receive the greater condemnation' (Jas. 3:1). A teacher who perceives one thought in his heart will sometimes utter ten. And what is even worse, he may sometimes utter ten, without perceiving even one. But perhaps it is true to say that in many cases this is done out of necessity, because of the nature of the ministry of spiritual fatherhood. He who speaks may or may not be inspired, but this is less important than that he trusts completely and unfailingly in Him Who performs all things.

Ultimately, however, we have only ourselves to blame if we do not live up to the spiritual measure of the saying in Wisdom of Jesus the son of Sirach, in imitation of the perfect hesychasm of the Mother of God. But when we begin to do so, we begin to taste of the sweetness of the fruits of hesychastic prayer, and then we do not want to occupy ourselves with anything but the invocation of Christ's Name. His Name becomes our very breath; indeed, it becomes even more vital to us than our breath, as St. John Chrysostom says: we need to breathe in order to sustain our physical life, but how much more do we need to invoke the Name in order to receive divine life?

I began by saying that God has perfected a Body in history. We need to invest everything of ourselves in this Body, His Church. Let those who can, do so through inner prayer, because this is very precious in the eyes of the Lord; let those who can, do so through bodily labour, not sparing themselves. They may perhaps do less than the others, but that is none the less useful in the building up of the Body of the Church, even as it is pleasing to God. Everything we invest in the building up, in the perfecting of this Body, makes us partakers of the glory that will be revealed at the end of time; everything we do is an investment in the eternal kingdom, and the investment of one member of the Body becomes a common inheritance for all the other members. As St. Basil the Great says, the gifts of one become the treasure of all.[10] 'And the multitude of them that believed were of one heart and of one soul: neither said any of them that aught of the things which he possessed was his own; but they had all things common,' says the Book of Acts (Acts 4:32). The Apostles invested everything they had in the Body, even their physical strength, and such was their desire that 'in singleness of heart' (ὁμοθυμαδόν) they waited upon the coming of the Lord, invoking the Name and breaking bread (cf. Acts 2:42, 46), that is to say, performing the Divine Liturgy. Ὁμοθυμαδόν means with one θυμός, that is, with one desire, one will, one heart.

Allow me to conclude by quoting one more passage from Fr. Sophrony's book *We Shall See Him as He Is,* where he speaks about spiritual life as the work of grace in us rather than the result of our own efforts, which are an abomination before God when we put our trust in them.

If the ascetic struggle be interpreted as the determined surmounting of our evil inclinations, then the life that is truly blessed with grace knows no struggle. The advent within a man of divine strength means that everything he does becomes a positive act, free of all inner contradictions. Both mind and heart, inspired by the love of Christ, are immune from doubt. When love of God is in full flood, it is transposed into contemplation of the uncreated Light, which removes passion and brings the unutterable delight of liberty of spirit, since man now dwells beyond death and fear.[11]

The aim of our spiritual fight is to overcome our common enemy – death,[12] and thereby gain eternal life. According to Fr. Sophrony, when man becomes a vessel of divine inspiration, his every act has a positive outcome (cf. Ps. 1:3) and is free of all inner contradiction. The grace of God has swallowed up all evil. Let us all heed the word of the Apostle: 'Be not overcome of evil, but overcome evil with good' (Rom. 12:21).

NOTES

1. *Cf. Saint Silouan, op. cit.,* p. 300.

2. *Cf.* St. Gregory Palamas, in *The Triads, op. cit.,* p. 43.

3. *Cf.* St. Maximus the Confessor, 'On the Lord's Prayer', in *The Philokalia,* Vol. 2 (London: Faber & Faber, 1981), p. 297.

4. 'To the Most Reverend Nun Xenia', in *The Philokalia*, *op. cit.*, p. 316.

5. *On Prayer, op. cit.*, p. 14.

6. *Ibid.*, p. 10.

7. *Ibid.*

8. *Ibid.*

9. *Ibid.*, p. 128.

10. *The Longer Rules* VII, in *The Ascetic Works of Saint Basil,* trans. W.K.L. Clarke (London: SPCK, 1925), p. 164.

11. *We Shall See Him as He Is, op. cit.*, p. 162.

12. *Ibid.*, p. 99.

CHAPTER FOURTEEN

THE WORD OF GOD
DIVINE INSPIRATION AND
PROPHETIC LIFE

CREATED IN THE IMAGE and likeness of God, man's existence is in no sense static. He is a dynamic personal being, and his calling is one of continual enlargement, according to the 'increase of God' (Col. 2:19). Inspiration for the realisation of this extraordinarily high calling is drawn from his encounter with the living word of God, and from his acceptance of it.

The word of God, spoken through His Son and in the power of His Spirit, is 'that inconceivable, infinite force that summoned from the darkness of non-existence into the light of life all that exists, the countless number of worlds, all the incalculable diversity of reasonable and non-reasonable beings.'[1] This same word reached Adam and Eve in a direct and immediate manner, providing them with an example of life, and a vision of eternity to orientate and guide them in their ways.

After the fall, during the Old Testament period, each time the word of God came to the prophets and resounded in their hearts, the event would unfailingly produce a transformation, making known upon earth the ways of the Most High in preparation for His advent in the flesh.

And when, finally, He did come in the form of our nature, the Son and Word of God showed that He Himself, He Who fashioned our hearts in the beginning (cf. Ps. 33:15), did so with a view to His coming, and in a manner appropriate to His evangelical teaching by which He offered us a way of restoration and regeneration.

Father Sophrony has a very beautiful word on the feast of the Transfiguration. He says that the Lord, before showing His glory to His disciples, neither spoke nor performed any miracles for one whole week, but remained in prayer together with them.[2] His aim was to show them that the revelation of God is given when the spirit of man prays in 'silence' (hesychia) in the Spirit of God. The Holy Fathers say that Christ Himself was born in the silence of the unoriginate Father. The Mother of God received the revelation of the gospel even as she lived in hesychia inside the Holy of Holies, practising the prayer of the heart. Moses fasted for forty days before entering into the cloud of God, which represents the glory of God. When Joshua laid siege to Jericho, he commanded the Israelites to do nothing but remain in hesychia for seven days; on the seventh day, the trumpets blew and the walls of Jericho fell by themselves (cf. Josh. ch. 6). There are plenty of examples in the scriptures which show that every creative word is preceded by hesychia. The conclusion to be drawn is that we must first find our heart through hesychia for the word of God to be born there.

Whenever the Word of God addressed the heart of man – before His Incarnation, in times of old, and also in the latter times, in the flesh – however brief His pronouncement may have been, it was holy and salutary because the mystery of the Cross was prophetically at work within His every utterance. It also revealed the kingdom of God, and the state of the fallen world, which stand as far from one another as the East does from the West, and as heaven does from earth.

The word of God is exceedingly great, but never terrifying in its visitation. Covered with the veil of humility, it cannot easily be comprehended, except in the measure of one's own humility, which opens the heart. We can only babble and stammer for in its true nature it remains indescribable. Nevertheless, when the heart opens wide to conceive and bear it in travail and pain, then a prophetic event takes place: God Himself enters into a life-long covenant with the soul, and she then becomes 'like them that dream' (Ps. 126:1), and her cup overflows with divine comfort (cf. Ps. 23:5). God invades the heart and grants the soul to be 'born again, not of corruptible seed, but of incorruptible, by the word of God, which liveth and abideth forever' (1 Pet. 1:23). This rebirth of the soul through the 'word of truth' (Eph. 1:13) is the defining experience of her contact with living eternity, and thereafter becomes the source of divine inspiration.

What we have just described is an event and the means by which God reveals Himself to man. As our Elder said, 'God speaks in brief *dicta* but life is not long enough to uncover their full content.'[3] The living word of God which so briefly visits man is loaded with eternity and gives a sense of the absolute character of knowledge of the divine. Again, in the words of our Elder, 'The divine word introduces a new, especial sense of being into the soul. The heart experiences a surge of light-bearing life. The mind suddenly grasps hitherto concealed meanings. Contact with His creative energy recreates us. Cognition that comes in this fashion is not the same as philosophical intellection: together with perception of realities of the spiritual plane man's whole being takes on another form of life – similar perhaps to the first-created. This existential knowledge of God dissolves into a current of prayerful love for Him.'[4]

This new existential knowledge of God is the 'light of life', about which the beginning of the fourth Gospel speaks. The experience and taste of it endow the soul with the wisdom to discern between uncreated energy or the incorruptible grace of God, and the created, mortal and corruptible nature of man. This knowledge provokes in us an ardent desire for the former, which involves the painful detachment from the latter, and the heart melts into prayerful love for God. These two elements – the wisdom of discernment that enlightens the mind, on the one hand, and the stirring of the heart to insatiable love of God, on the other – constitute something which may be defined as divine inspiration. To put it another way, the combination of these two factors consumes the spirit of the man in whom divine inspiration is present.

The inspiration of God in man begets a certain quality, a certain disposition of his spirit. According to the definition of our Elder, 'inspiration is the presence of the power of the Holy Spirit within us'.[5] This charismatic presence of Christ in us directs all those things that we subject to it towards a certain purpose – the divinisation of the entire being. In other words, inspiration purifies everything that is susceptible to purification – the body and all the powers of the soul. It consumes every impurity of the mind and casts away all those things that resist the breath of the Holy Spirit. At times, as St. Paul says, it takes the form of 'a certain fearful looking for of judgment and fiery indignation, which shall devour the adversaries' (Heb. 10:27).

But inspiration is also an ardent desire which disposes the heart to struggle intensely for the preservation of that dynamic faith which, as St. Paul says, 'worketh by love' (Gal. 5:6). In his account of the life of St. Anthony the Great, St. Athanasius the Great says that it was by the intensity of his desire that the saint measured his progress, and not by the length of time for which he had dwelt in the desert. And he preserved this intensity by forgetting the past and making a new beginning every day, applying to himself the saying of St. Paul: 'This one thing I do, forgetting those things which are behind, and reaching forth unto those things which are before, I press toward the mark for the prize of the high calling of God in Christ Jesus' (Phil. 3:13–14). He remembered also the words of the Prophet Elijah who said, 'The Lord of hosts liveth, before whom I stand . . . today' (1 Kgs. 18:15). This expresses the desire and the readiness of the prophet to obey the will of God at every moment. But should man find himself lacking in such ardour and inspiration, he can hardly avoid being a servant of 'the religion of his own will', in Greek, ἐθελοθρησκία (cf. Col. 2:23). Then he is full and he is rich (cf. 1 Cor. 4:8); he lives an illusion 'after the tradition of men, after the rudiments of the world, and not after Christ' (Col. 2:8).

As we have said, man is a dynamic being. When he is inspired, he becomes possessed of a blessed *élan*. As the Psalmist says, 'I will run the way of Thy commandments when Thou shalt enlarge my heart' (Ps. 119:32). This enlargement of the heart provokes in him a hunger and thirst after God's righteousness (*cf.* Matt. 5:6). The heart of man becomes as a 'dry and thirsty land' (Ps. 63:1), and his thirst can be quenched only by the Holy Spirit, the 'well of water springing up into everlasting life', as the Lord said (John 4:14).

Divine inspiration keeps man continuously in the presence of God. He yearns for an ever greater fullness of this presence that now pervades him. He is possessed of the same determination as was the Prophet David when he said, 'I will not give sleep to mine eyes, or slumber to mine eyelids, until I find out a place for the Lord, an habitation for the mighty God of Jacob' (Ps. 132:4–5). Such perfect inspiration can be likened to the state of the angels who 'rest not day and night, saying, Holy, Holy, Holy, Lord God Almighty, which was, and is, and is to come' (Rev. 4:8).

However, inspiration in our present state has a 'cruel' side, for love, its main constituent, can be no less than utterly demanding. Solomon expressed this truth in a wonderful way when he said, 'Love is strong as death. . . . Many waters cannot quench love, neither can the floods drown it; if a man would give all the substance of his house for love, it would utterly be contemned' (Song 8:6–7). Indeed, man remains an unprofitable servant to the end (*cf.* Luke 17:10). We note, however, that Solomon lived at a time when death still had dominion, and that, according to the New Testament, love is stronger than death.

We read in the Acts of the Apostles that in this world Christ 'should suffer' (Acts 26:23). He is indeed one who 'suffers' (παθητός), for such is His love. God offers man His boundless love, which is the great and needful 'good part' referred to by the Lord when He spoke to Martha (*cf.* Luke 10:42); and man, in his turn, offers God his heart as a 'tiny part'. Man suffers because his heart is so infinitesimal, whereas 'God is greater than his heart' (1 John 3:20). Man is therefore condemned by his own heart, which is unable to contain the fullness of divine love. This produces a great tension in the man who would join his 'tiny part' to God's 'great part'. For example, a prophet is inspired and led by the Holy Spirit, and therefore suffers the torment of this tension until he becomes a 'temple of the living God' (2 Cor. 6:16). He suffers for the sake of God: he is unable to contain Him, and he will not find rest until he becomes His habitation. He suffers also for his fellows, desiring that all be pure and spotless brides of Christ, that Christ be formed in their hearts.

Divine inspiration produces in us the desire to rid our heart of every stain, that it may be overshadowed by the light of the Great Visitor. There is godly zeal in this desire, and the Lord Himself was consumed with the same zeal when He went up to Jerusalem to cleanse God's house (cf. John 2:17), and we are called to imitate Him in this. As the Lord said, 'I am come to send fire on the earth; and what will I, if it be already kindled?' (Luke 12:49).

We have said that prophetic life consists of bearing divine inspiration and being moved by the Holy Spirit. This is confirmed by St. Peter, who said that the Apostles were 'holy men of God who spake as they were moved by the Holy Ghost' (2 Pet. 1:21). We, too, must never forget that 'one is our Master, even Christ' (Matt. 23:10). He is the supreme Prophet, for He came in the flesh as the 'Forerunner' of His spiritual and glorious second coming. By word and deed He taught us the way, that we too might change from the carnal to the spiritual. His great desire was to prepare us, that we might be worthy of beholding His divinity which will be fully revealed at the end of time.

This prophetic Way of Christ is described by St. Paul: 'When He ascended up on high, He led captivity captive, and gave gifts to men. Now that He ascended, what is it but that He also descended first into the lower parts of the earth? He that descended is the same also that ascended up far above all heavens, that He might fill all things' (Eph. 4:8–10). The descent of Christ into the lower parts of the earth, that is, to hell, is in fact the source of every spiritual gift. And we too must go downwards if we are to know true prophetic life and be moved by the Holy Spirit. Men want thrones – they want to go up. This is the mind and tendency of the fallen world, but the Lord's path goes downward.

In his book on St. Silouan, Fr. Sophrony explains this downward movement. He says that the whole of humanity forms a pyramid. At its apex are seated the princes of this world who exercise authority over the nations (*cf.* Matt. 20:25); but in fact the spirit of man aspires to that primordial equality and justice which prevailed in Paradise before the fall. And the Lord has honoured this aspiration of man, for He inverted the pyramid and placed Himself at its apex, which was now its lowest point. He has thereby taken upon Himself the sins and the weight of all humanity and, in so doing, He has restored all things and has provided a most excellent way to attain to whatsoever things are true, honest, just, pure, lovely (*cf.* Phil. 4:8) and, therefore, salutary. Thus did Christ institute the supreme perfection (which is the essence of His Spirit) for the sake of man. 'The Son of man came not to be ministered unto, but to minister, and to give his life a ransom for many' (Matt. 20:28). In tracing the path for us, Christ went down, lower down than anyone else has ever been, and was 'made a curse for us' (Gal. 3:13). And all those who follow Him take the same route; they go down to meet with the Head of the inverted pyramid, for they cannot rest unless they be united with Him. Fr. Sophrony puts it this way: 'At the base of the overturned pyramid – the unfathomable base which is really the summit – is He Who took upon Himself the sins and burdens of the world, the Christ crucified in love for the world. And there we remark a quite especial life, a quite especial light, an especial fragrance. This is where love attracts the athletes of Christ.'[6] And this is prophetic life: to be possessed by this attraction to go down.

The following of Christ's downward path is accompanied by a twofold vision, a double consciousness. Firstly, the soul beholds Christ's example, of which the Lord spoke during the Last Supper. She contemplates Christ's ascent to Golgotha, His offering of His life, His acceptance of the death by which mankind was stricken, and His gift of divine life; and all this according to His words: 'This is my commandment, that ye love one another, as I have loved you . . .

for all things that I have heard of my Father I have made known unto you' (John 15:12, 15). In Gethsemane, the Lord prays for the whole Adam. He goes up to Golgotha alone, bearing in His heart the whole of humankind. He takes upon Himself the sins of the world. He delivers Himself up to extreme suffering for the sake of our release from the tyranny of the enemy, which weighs so heavily upon the whole of humanity because of the original sin in Paradise. He bears within Himself the whole Adam, all the peoples of all times, and then He dies for them all. No mortal could have assisted Him in any way. In the description in the Gospel, we see that His entire mind was united to His Father. He offered His life in order to receive that death by which humankind was stricken. And then, at His rising from the dead, He bears the content of His prayer, of His love and His determination, for with Him arises the whole Adam.

When we contemplate the holiness and humble love of Christ-God, the soul is so astounded and the heart so warmed that in his deep veneration man can only worship Him with gratitude and love. But in the light of this contemplation and experience, man sees his own untruth. According to Fr. Sophrony, 'The heart . . . beholds Christ's love embracing the whole of creation in infinite compassion for all that exists. . . . This vision moves the soul, astonishes the mind. Involuntarily we bow before Him. And however much we try to become like Him in humility, we do not attain to Him.'[7]

This twofold vision of God's infinite and humble love, on the one hand, and our unworthiness and incapacity for it, on the other, is an indispensable precondition for our dynamic increase in God, which is the purpose of our life. Indeed, this twofold vision is a prophetic state, a spiritual miracle. Fr. Sophrony describes this state repeatedly. He says, 'The more I "see" God, the more ardent does my repentance become, since I the more clearly recognise my unworthiness in His sight.'[8] In another place, he emphasises our need for this twofold vision: 'I must see Christ "as He Is" in order to confront myself with Him and thus perceive my "deformity". I cannot know myself unless I have His Holy Image before me.'[9] He also says that this double consciousness stirs up in us inspiration and gratitude to God our Benefactor. 'But', he acknowledges, 'here lies a paradox, a twofold consciousness in me, of my own nothingness, which I find abhorrent, and, on the other hand, of the compassionate condescendence of God.'[10]

With this tension in mind, we also remember St. John the Baptist, and his prophetic attitude towards his Master: 'He must increase, but I must decrease' (John 3:30). The Forerunner speaks here of their respective glory. We consider also the case of Isaiah the Prophet of the Old Testament, who relates his vision as follows: 'I saw also the Lord sitting upon a throne, high and lifted up. . . . Above it stood the Seraphim. . . . And the one cried unto the other, and said, Holy, Holy, Holy, is the Lord of hosts: the whole earth is full of His glory. . . . Then said I, Woe is me! for I am undone; because I am a man of unclean lips . . . for mine eyes have seen the King, the Lord of hosts. Then flew one of the Seraphim unto me, having a live coal in his hand, which he had taken with the tongs from off the altar and he laid it upon my mouth, and said, Lo, this hath touched thy lips, and thine iniquity is taken away, and thy sin is purged' (Isa. 6:1–7).

This twofold vision or double consciousness renders man prophetic and therefore truthful. Furthermore, this is the only situation in which his truthfulness is infallible. Listen to St. John the Divine: 'If we say that we have no sin, we deceive ourselves and the truth is not in us. If we confess our sins, He is faithful and just to forgive us our sins, and to cleanse us from all unrighteousness. If we say that we have not sinned, we make Him a liar, and His word is not in us' (1 John 1:8–10). And, of course, when we are made truthful, we attract the Spirit of Truth, the Spirit of Christ. We now confess the truth of the cosmic event of Adam's fall. We acknowledge also the supracosmic event of Christ's redemption. We bear witness to the eternal truth of His first coming in the flesh. We likewise bear witness to and anticipate His Second Coming in glory. We become His prophets for His word has been conceived in our hearts, firstly for our own salvation, and then for the salvation of the whole world through God's grace and lovingkindness.

NOTES

1. *Saint Silouan, op. cit.,* p. 214.

2. *Cf.* Archimandrite Sophrony, Ἄσκησις καὶ Θεωρία, *op. cit.,* p 180.

3. *On Prayer, op. cit.,* p. 38.

4. *Ibid.,* p. 35.

5. *We Shall See Him as He Is, op. cit.,* p. 119.

6. *Saint Silouan, op. cit.,* p. 239.

7. *On Prayer, op. cit.,* p. 14.

8. *We Shall See Him as He Is, op. cit.,* p. 152.

9. *Ibid.,* p. 59.

10. *Ibid.,* p. 180.

CHAPTER FIFTEEN

ON THE GIFT OF SPEAKING IN TONGUES[1]

TEN DAYS AFTER THE LORD'S ASCENSION into heaven, the gifts of the Holy Spirit were manifested on the day of Pentecost as a sign of the reconciliation that had occurred between God and man. But one of these gifts in particular, that of speaking in tongues, was different. The gift is a difficult one to understand, partly because it had all but disappeared by the end of the life of the Holy Apostle Paul. Moreover, it is clear from the later epistles of St. Paul, in which he puts it last on the list of the gifts of the Holy Spirit, that its importance had diminished. How are we to understand this?

We know that the gift of speaking in tongues (*glossolalia*) was given to the nascent Church for a specific purpose. The old Israel had become accustomed to worshipping and praying in a largely external manner, and when the Spirit came on the day of Pentecost, He wanted this to change. His intention, therefore, was to teach the people to pray in spirit, in the 'hidden man of the heart' (1 Pet. 3:4). But on the day of Pentecost, we see that the people began to speak in foreign tongues of the mighty works of God; the gift was soon widespread, because God wanted His words to go 'unto the ends of the world' (Rom. 10:18) and the new faith to bring salvation to all the peoples. Many were encouraged to speak in tongues, and the Spirit of God condescended accordingly. Those who prayed in tongues were happy, being certain of one thing: God 'had broken into' them and was at work within them.

However, this gift slowly began to disappear, for it would no longer be useful or helpful in the edification of the Body. It often happened that glorifications and words would be pronounced which the Body itself could not understand, and this would require the help of an interpreter inspired by the Holy Spirit. Although some of the faithful continued to use their gifts of tongues, at some point it became clear that the prayer of those who were listening was no longer being inspired in the same way as before. For this reason, St. Paul says the following in the Epistle to the Corinthians: 'I will pray with the spirit, and I will pray with the understanding also: I will sing with the spirit, and I will sing with the understanding also' (1 Cor. 14:15). Thus, he distinguishes between prayer in the spirit (*pneuma*) and prayer in the mind (*nous*), and identifies prayer in the spirit with praying in foreign tongues. One verse earlier he says, 'If I pray in an unknown tongue, my spirit prayeth, but my understanding is unfruitful' (1 Cor. 14:14).

It is true that for St. Paul, spirit and mind are almost identical: he sometimes says that the highest purpose of Christianity is the renewal of the spirit and sometimes the renewal of the *nous*. Nevertheless, in trying to distinguish between the two, I would say that the spirit is present in the mind as something higher, deeper than the mind itself – that it is revealed through the mind, just as the soul can be said to be revealed through the emotions.

But when the Holy Apostle says 'I will pray with the spirit, and I will pray with the understanding also', we must admit that a certain opposition has been introduced. Prayer in the spirit is identified with prayer in tongues, when man's spirit is aware of the irruption of God into his life. Furthermore, there were times when the grace that taught the people to worship God 'in spirit and truth' (John 4:2) – with their inner being – was present in such abundance that it flowed out in torrents of enthusiasm. In this kind of prayer the highest faculty of the human being is inspired by God, receiving His energy. Man then surrenders to the 'breath' of the Holy Spirit, which 'bloweth where it listeth' (John 3:8), and the Spirit intercedes with 'unutterable groanings' (Rom. 8:26) for those in whom He dwells, sometimes with words which are beyond the understanding of the psychological man.

In prayer of the mind, by contrast, the mind rises towards God in pious thought and godly desire. Such prayer is characterised by holy contrition or joy, but it is not liable to surrender to the great impetus and boundless spiritual exaltation we have just described. A degree of control is exercised by the person who prays in the mind: he is able to direct his thoughts, desires and feelings. His spiritual faculties act in the usual way, in characteristic order; his prayers and doxologies are pronounced in an altogether understandable manner, and can provoke any hearers to participation in the worship. Of course, the heart participates in this kind of prayer of the mind, but there is a definite absence of total surrender to the breath of the Spirit. St. Paul recommends both types of prayer. He advises us not to use either one to the exclusion of the other, considering that it may at times be better to pray in tongues, and at others with the mind. When we pray in the spirit, we pray for ourselves and for God, but when we pray in the mind, we pray not only for God and for ourselves, but also for the edification of our neighbour and, therefore, for the rest of the Body.

It is, however, surprising to see that St. Paul shows a definite preference for prayer of the mind, which is a free activity of the human spirit, rather than for prayer of the spirit, which is a pure gift of the Holy Spirit. But his choice is entirely in keeping with the rest of the Epistle to the Corinthians. For example, he also says that the true prophet will be in control of his spirit: 'The spirits of the prophets are subject to the prophets' (1 Cor 14:32). Total surrender to *glossolalia* involves a certain loss of control: it is an explosion of grace and joy, and while we are fully aware that God is within us, somehow we deny ourselves any awareness of our fellow-members of the Body.

Many in the early Church were gifted with tongues, but over time the gift became rarer. The problem was, quite simply, that if someone spoke in tongues, he would unintentionally take up all the spiritual space of the congregation as a whole, which would not derive the least profit from the gift. The best explanation for God's gift of tongues to the early Church lies in the necessity of teaching newly-converted Christians to pray with their heart rather than just externally, as they were likely to have been used to doing. But the Church soon discovered a deeper way to educate the heart, for She was concerned to cultivate the inner man. She discovered the invocation of the Name of our Lord Jesus Christ. And little by little, the Prayer of the Heart replaced the gift of speaking in tongues. The Jesus Prayer is a way of praying in the spirit without losing any control of the spirit, and, therefore, without running the risk of usurping the space of the other members of the Body of Christ. (All the things we do in church must be done in a way that respects the spiritual space of our fellows. When I was studying theology in Paris, I learned from my old professors that the priest could sometimes lift up his hands in the Divine Liturgy, but also that there is an unwritten rule that he should not lift them above the level of his ears. Similarly, with the Gospel and the censer or when we say, 'The Holy things unto the holy', we take care not to exaggerate our movements. We must be humble and discreet, so that our behaviour does not attract the attention of the others.)

In conclusion, to speak in tongues or to pray in the spirit is indeed to immerse our *nous* in the sea of the Spirit. But the Apostle himself prefers to draw us in to shore, that we avoid even the possibility of disorder in the Body of the Church, and that everything be done for the sake of the edification of the people.

By far, the best possible way of approaching the phenomenon of *glossolalia* in our times, as our Tradition teaches us to understand it – that is, without condemning or criticising – is to consider that, if people are prevented from worshipping God with the heart, God can once again bestow on them this gift of speaking in tongues. The fact that this gift has reappeared now in modern times, when the way of the heart has been forgotten or is not known, points towards one single purpose. Clearly, the Spirit of God yearns to lead all people home to the Church, to place them within the Body of the Church, and to instruct them in this noble form of worship that has been practised by Christians for so many centuries, that their hearts might once more be cultivated through the invocation of the Name of our Lord Jesus Christ. And we know that whosoever bears His Name, does so unto salvation, 'for there is none other name under heaven given among men, whereby we must be saved' (Acts 4:12). If this gift has indeed been given temporarily to some people, perhaps it will enable them to discover the true unbroken Tradition of the Church, the Tradition of the Prayer of the Heart, which is the surest and humblest prayer in the edification, inspiration and salvation of man. Through this prayer, we receive the greatest of all the gifts of the Holy Spirit, the gift which will heal our nature and strengthen it, 'guiding us into all truth' (John 16:13). It will enable us to bear the fullness of divine love. And this gift will never outlive its purpose – indeed, it will accompany us beyond the grave.

It is important that we understand this phenomenon of *glossolalia* – we must not be seduced by it. But let us, above all, be gracious to those who believe they have experienced this gift, and gently point out to them that it is the beginning of something far greater that will lead them to the heart of the Tradition. In order to evangelise people, we will not reject them, or dismiss them as 'heretics'. We will rather try to find a positive element, and use it to lead them to the full truth, as St. Paul did when he addressed the Athenians. He used their 'unknown God' (Acts 17:23) to lead them to the One True God, the known and beloved God.

QUESTIONS AND ANSWERS

Question 1: What is the connection between language and speaking in tongues at Pentecost, when the Holy Spirit came upon the Apostles?

Answer 1: At Pentecost, they spoke in different languages. They were Parthians, Medes, Elamites, etc., and those who received the gift spoke in those tongues, but in their exaltation, they also spoke in unknown tongues. The Apostle Paul says that they themselves did not understand what they were saying and needed someone else to interpret. But where is the benefit in that? They know that they worship God, but the others receive no profit. Of course, there have been occasions in the history of the Church when holy people received this gift and were able to communicate through it; for example, when St. Basil the Great and St. Ephraim the Syrian met, neither of them knew the other's language, but they managed to understand each other.

Question 2: Currently in America, among the Pentecostals and the Charismatics, there is a certain contention that speaking in tongues is some secret prayer-language provided to them by God, through the Holy Spirit, such that the devil cannot snatch away their prayers. Could you comment on that?

Answer 2: Maybe what these people feel is real, but what they say is wrong. Sometimes people do not understand what they go through. Maybe they have received a touch of the Spirit, because God looks at the heart of man, but when they start speaking, they make mistakes, because they do not have the key to interpret their experiences, and the key is the Tradition. In the West, I have often seen people receiving great gifts. There was a minister in a town south of London, and when he preached you thought that honey was running from his mouth. I happened to hear some tapes of his talks. He had such a gift and mind for the Scriptures! With such ease he used to combine different parts of the Scriptures, using one passage to speak for the other, and it was such a pleasure and joy to listen to him! He had this gift for a certain time in his evangelical parish, but suddenly the thought came to him that he must go out and preach the word of God to the whole world. Unfortunately, he had no point of reference in his church, no one to discern the will of God for him, and tell him, 'No, God has put you in this place. Stay here! It seems that the Spirit bears witness that this is your place.' Anyway, he embraced the idea of going and preaching the Gospel to the whole world, and after a few years, I happened to hear that he was in Switzerland in a state of depression, not even wanting to celebrate the Lord's Supper. He would ask a layman to do it, while he would just sit in a corner, downhearted. I think that he had this great gift for a certain time, but there was no Tradition to uphold and strengthen him, or to help him discern the ways of salvation and of the Spirit. Consequently, when the moment of trial came, he was lost. The problem these people face is that there is no institution of the Church, because there is no Tradition. There are individuals who sometimes, because of their personal love for God and the Scriptures, have a certain enthusiasm and they manage to do a lot, but it all evaporates so easily, because there is no vessel in which to place and store the grace that they have received. For us the vessel is the institution of the Church, together with the Tradition which is the vehicle that carries us. I do not despise them – some of them are very gifted people – but they are the victims of their own traditions. There is no stability in them, because they have no notion of the Church in the sense that we do. We often have Anglican priests visiting our monastery, and they keep saying to us, 'Only you, the Orthodox, have an unbroken Tradition.' But they say no more, they do not go any further and, of course, I keep quiet. What can you say?

Question 3: Some years ago, I heard a *theologumenon* for the gift of speaking in tongues, and I would like your reaction. It said that the original gift continued Pentecost and used the languages of humanity, and that when the languages of humanity had all been covered, the gift ended.

Answer 3: Yes, it implies the idea that the gift of *glossolalia* was given just to bless all our languages. I think I have read something similar in St. John Chrysostom, but I do not remember it exactly. Nevertheless, whoever has the experience of the true Tradition of the Orthodox Church has no want, he lacks nothing. All the modern Christian denominations reflect certain aspects of our Tradition. They call themselves Evangelicals, but surely we are evangelical too, maybe even more than they are.

Question 4: Either someone gave me, or I purchased a copy of the spiritual memoirs of Elder Porphyrios, called *Wounded by Love.* I began to read it, and he describes how he received the gift of the Holy Spirit of clear sight. He was praying in the narthex of the church, when an old hermit came into the church. Thinking he was alone, the hermit spread his arms out like a cross and made sounds that could be described as *glossolalia,* and he became radiant with the light of God. Fr. Porphyrios, from that moment, believed that his gift of clear sight was connected with the prayer of the old hermit. So the process of receiving the gift was very hidden and secret. My question is, are there any other similar things we find in our Tradition?

Answer 4: All of us more or less know something of the gift of speaking in tongues, or praying in spirit. When we are alone in our rooms, we pray in ways in which we cannot pray in church, in front of others. We can just let ourselves be immersed in the Spirit of God and speak to Him in an unrestrained way. We can say to Him, 'Lord, I thank Thee that Thou art as Thou art and there is none like Thee', or 'Lord, it would be better not to live even one day upon earth than to be without Thy love.' When the Spirit carries us in that way, we utter prayers which are very personal, and we feel the power of the Spirit within, but in no way could we pray in like manner together with our brethren. That is why we read in a neutral tone in church, so that the others who are there can listen to the reading if they want to, or if they do not want to, they can follow their inner rhythm of prayer without being disturbed. It is unacceptable to read in a sentimental, personal way in church, because it undermines the peace of others. I have heard readings which were really awful; I could not bear it, and I just wanted to run away from the church. Sometimes, in monasteries, monks appear to read in a manner that may even seem impious, just flat and straight, because they know that other monks might have spent the whole night in prayer in their cells, and have come to church with all their spirit recollected in their heart, so they just want to keep the same rhythm of prayer. And this is possible as long as everything in church is done in a neutral way.

We even try to understand the gift of speaking in tongues in the same spirit. Maybe God gives this gift in order to help people to learn to pray with their heart, to make the transition from the external to the inner. I am sure many of you have known this kind of prayer. Many times, when you are in your room, and God gives a particular grace and inspiration, you can kneel down, you can knock your head on the floor, you can beat your chest, you can do whatever you like, but when you are in the church, you do not usurp the space of your fellows. What a great culture! I remember a story from the Desert Fathers. A great old man of the desert of Egypt entered the church and, thinking that he was alone, he let a big sigh come out of him unrestrained. Suddenly he heard some movement in a corner and realised that there was a novice hidden in the church, praying. He went and prostrated to him and said to him, 'Forgive me brother, for I have not yet made a beginning.'[2]

Many of the Desert Fathers had this culture of hiding their charisms. One great ascetic received three monks in his cell. He wanted to observe their practice, so he pretended to be asleep. The three monks, thinking that their host was sleeping, encouraged each other, and then started praying. He saw the prayer of two of them coming out like a flame, while the third one prayed with difficulty. But they had waited for their host to fall asleep and they had themselves pretended to be asleep, so that everything could be done in secret, without losing the reward of our Father Who sees in secret and rewards openly. Every precaution is taken so as not to lose the ethos of humility. This is the great culture of the Orthodox Church, and we must not lose it!

Question 5: There are three places in the New Testament that record Jesus speaking in Aramaic: 'Eli, Eli, lama sabachthani', 'Talitha cumi', and 'Abba (Father)'. Why didn't the New Testament authors translate into Greek or Hebrew these words that Jesus spoke? Are there any written commentaries or reflections on the usage of the Aramaic?

Answer 5: I do not really know how to answer your question, but perhaps the fact that these sayings were recorded in that dialect preserved their full impact and meaning. Looking at translations of the New Testament from the original Greek, I see that in many cases the text does not make any sense, although those who translated the New Testament into English or French were great scholars. I have in mind, for example, 2 Corinthians 5:8-10; I have not found any translation that is able to render the Greek meaning. The West is a victim of bad translations. Probably, when the Evangelists wanted to have a particular impact, they used Aramaic, but they could not use too much, because then they would have written the whole Gospel in that dialect. But there may be other reasons. My answer reflects my own preoccupation – I think I am a bit prejudiced against bad translations!

Question 6: Concerning the previous question, the way it was presented suggests that the text was originally written in Greek. It was not written in Greek; all the Gospels circulated originally in Aramaic and were translated into Greek later. 'Eli, Eli, lama sabachthani' was recorded in Aramaic, because of the implication of the language Jesus used, meaning that He was calling His God. If you put the same words into Greek or any other language, the same meaning would not be rendered. There is no meaning once you translate it.

Answer 6: But there the Gospel also gives the translation into Greek. It keeps the original dialect, but immediately it also gives the translation, maybe to avoid the kind of confusion that had existed among the people. When they heard these words, they thought that Jesus, at that moment, was calling Elijah. I am not a scholar and I do not know, but I find it difficult to admit that St. Luke's Gospel was written in Aramaic.

A Brief Comment: Many years ago, I met an Orthodox priest who had led his entire congregation into the whole speaking-in-tongues 'thing' and then, eventually, led his whole congregation back out of it. A man, who had become Orthodox, came to him and said, 'You know, I speak in tongues regularly.' And this priest asked him to do one thing: 'The next time you speak in tongues, make the sign of the cross over your mouth and see what happens.' The man did so and, as he related the story, thirty days later he realised he had not spoken in tongues, not even once. He decided to speak again, and once more he made the sign of the cross over his mouth. A full year went by before he realised again that he had not spoken in tongues. Then he decided to try it one more time; again he made the sign of the cross over his mouth. He never spoke in tongues again for the rest of his life.

Question 7: You said several times during the last couple of days that we should use the Jesus Prayer as a way to assist us. But at one time in Russia, they had to forbid people from using the Jesus Prayer because they were using it like a magic incantation. Could you comment on how that happens?

Answer 7: I have heard about this matter, but I have not studied it. What I know is that when there are no transgressions, the law is not needed. The law appears only when there are transgressions. Therefore, for as long as we use what the Church gives us properly, there is no need for any prohibition, but when there are deviations, then the Church has to take measures.

Question 8: On a number of occasions, you have made the distinction between the spiritual and the psychological reality: spiritual tears versus psychological tears, spiritual grief and shame versus psychological grief and shame. That distinction has been very helpful to me and I think to others as well. Do you think there is also a psychological use of the Jesus Prayer versus a deep spiritual use of it?

Answer 8: I do not know, but, of course, the Jesus Prayer can cover all the levels of human life. The energy that accompanies the Name of Christ, when it is invoked with reverence, humility and attention, is always spiritual, and, of course, it will satisfy all the needs of the person. If it satisfies the spiritual needs of the person, surely it will also satisfy the psychological ones, and will bring peace even to the body. There are three levels of existence: the physical, the psychological and the spiritual. From the physical to the spiritual, the distance is the same in all people, but in women the middle level is a bit higher than for men, that is why sometimes women confuse psychological states with spiritual states. It is more difficult for men to confuse the two, but they are more vulnerable on the physical level. Women can stay longer on the psychological level, whereas men cannot; they fall too quickly on the carnal level. We priests specially must know that and always be on our guard. The distance between the ordinary level of life as we all live it, and the level of sanctification is the same for both male and female, but the distances between the three levels – physical, psychological and spiritual – is different in men and women. Fr. Sophrony explained this to us, and it is something useful to know in our pastoral care. It is good to know where our vulnerability lies, so that we are careful.

Question 9: My question is linked with the last thing that our Lord said on the Cross: 'It is completed' or 'finished.' Was the whole thing done prior to His death? Is the finished work separate from His death and Resurrection? How does salvation fit into all this and how do you understand the reversal of what happened in the Garden of Eden, the results of the sin of Adam and Eve, how they were expelled, how mankind has been under a curse ever since – and has the curse been removed?

Answer 9: 'It is finished' means 'It is perfected', because the sacrifice was accomplished by the death of the Lord. At that moment, the unjust death of the Lord, which was a condemnation of the just death we received because of our sin, was taking place. In the Garden of Gethsemane, the Lord prayed sweating drops of blood for the salvation of the world. The sacrifice in the spirit was already being offered then, but it was to be sealed with Christ's physical death on the Cross. Our death is a just death, because it is the result of our sins, but Christ's death was unjust, because He was sinless. But he voluntarily gave Himself to death in our place in order to destroy our death. And, of course, once the sacrifice was offered, everything was restored, it was enough for our salvation. I do not know if I understood exactly what you said.

Question 10: Through Christ's Cross and Resurrection salvation came, but do we have this experience in the Church?

Answer 10: We have it partly, and the saints even more fully. In this life, it is always in part, but this is a guarantee of the fullness to come after the General Resurrection. Now we receive the earnest of the spirit, the deposit of the capital which will be fully entrusted to us in that day. What is important for now is that we have the assurance and the information in our heart that this restoration has already taken place. Whether we have but a little warmth in our heart when we invoke the risen Lord, or a greater rapture by the Spirit, it is the same thing: they both testify to the same reality – that the Lord is risen and death has no more dominion.

He has conquered death and the world. Even when we have a little token of that life, which is to come fully in that day, it is enough to confirm us on our way. For 'he that is faithful in that which is least is faithful also in much: and he that is unjust in the least is unjust also in much' (Luke 16:10). We see this in the life of St. Peter: although the Lord had told him that he would deny Him thrice, he wanted to be courageous and did not measure his strength. When he entered the Praetorium to see how things would turn out, a little girl came to him saying, 'Oh, you are a Galilean; you are from the company of Jesus.' There was no danger, but maybe St. Peter despised the maiden and thought that she was not worthy to hear about the Prophet of Galilee. He was careless and said, 'I do not know what you are talking about.' So he slid a bit and the enemy found a little place to get a grip on him. After a little while, again the same remark, 'Ah, you too are of the company of the Galilean.' This time he slipped a bit further, and he replied, 'I do not know the man.' Then the enemy had even more of a grip on him. The third time he denied Christ and apostasised, that is to say, in a way he lost his baptism. He completely alienated himself from the Lord. Thank God that the Lord had prayed beforehand and that the energy of His prayer remained to save him! And when the cock crowed, and the Lord turned to him, Peter was wounded in the heart, he went out, and wept bitterly (Matt. 26:69–75). You see, because he was careless in a little thing, in the end the temptation was beyond his measure. It is the same with us: if we are not careful in little things, we fall in big things. For example, if someone comes and tells us, 'Let us go and rob a bank', we will rebuke him: 'Go away! What are you saying?' But maybe we will be careless enough to pocket five dollars that do not belong to us, but to the Church. Thus, we slip a bit; then the enemy has a grip on us, and we can go further and further and do worse things. Another example: if somebody comes and tells us, 'Let us go and fornicate!' we will reply, 'Go away! How could I defile the temple of God and make it an instrument of impurity?' But if we allow even a little familiarity with another person, then the enemy gets a grip on us and we go further, each time starting where we left off the previous time, and finally we sink into the mud of impurity. The words of Scripture work both ways: whoever is faithful in little will be given strength by God to acquire even that which is great; and whoever is not faithful or careful in little, and allows familiarity, injustice, or something else to creep into his life, will be found unfaithful in that which is great, and he will be completely lost. We see such things happening all the time in the life of the Church; therefore, it is better to be careful and keep the word of the Lord. Forgive me.

NOTES

1. My understanding of the gift of speaking in tongues is based on Fr. Sophrony's teachings, and on the ideas expressed by St. Philaret of Moscow in his sermon on 1 Cor. 14:15 ('I will pray with the spirit, and I will pray with the understanding also: I will sing with the spirit, and I will sing with the understanding also'), in *Choix de Sermons et Discours*, Vol. II, trans. A. Serpinet (Paris: E. Dentu, 1866), pp. 435–445.

2. Abba Tithoes in *The Sayings of the Desert Fathers, op. cit.*, p. 198; see also, *ibid.*, John the Dwarf, p. 77.

EPILOGUE

*Sermon for the Leave-taking of the Feast of the Meeting of Our Lord Jesus Christ in the Temple**

I T IS A JOY FOR ME to be in your midst again and to celebrate the Liturgy together, sustained by your prayers. It is very significant that it so happens that our Divine Liturgy should take place today, on the Leave-taking of the Presentation of the Lord in and to the Temple, for it is in fact also the feast of the royal priesthood of Christ.

The presentation of the Lord begins in the temple of God, and last time you invited me to your clergy retreat we spoke about the double presentation of Christ, before God and before men.[1] Christ justified men before God by His true and perfect example, and if we follow it we shall never be confounded, and we will be received by the Father and the Spirit and become sons of God. He also justified God before men because He loved us to the end, unto death, and worked our salvation in this manner. But His presentation is also the beginning of the manifestation of His priesthood, which is significant for us, because we are partakers of His priesthood. There is only one priesthood, the royal priesthood of the Lord, of which all Christians are partakers; but we, as ordained priests, are partakers in a double way.

I would like to stay my mind a little on those two people that were in the temple and who received Christ: St. Simeon, a man 'just and devout', as Scripture says, and the Prophetess Anna. Both were well-stricken in years, but they had a strong expectation in their heart of the redemption to come, and they awaited the incorruptible 'consolation of Israel', which was Christ (Luke 2:25). That is to say, they were constantly stirring up the prophetic gift in their hearts, having become partakers of God's prophetic Spirit.

Priesthood is also a prophetic gift, and we have to stir it up all the time and keep it alive to the end. We do this by ensuring that God's incorruptible consolation is always present in our heart. And when this consolation abounds in the heart, we are enabled to console others, the people of God, who come to us. These two people, Simeon and Anna, are examples of people who prophetically shared in the royal priesthood of Christ. Their expectation was great, and they awaited the consolation of Israel just as we, the people of God's New Israel, also await the great day of the Lord's coming again.

The Lord 'bowed the heavens and came down' (*cf.* Ps. 144:5), and His coming to us in the flesh is the prophecy of His Second Coming. Those, therefore, who have loved His appearing in our flesh live in great longing for His Second Coming in the glory of His Father; they do not simply live in expectation, they rather hasten towards His Second Coming – such is their desire to meet the Lord.

When the Lord came, He became the 'sign' of God for all generations which would be spoken against, as today's Gospel says (Luke 2:34). That is to say, there can be no neutrality in our attitude to Him. If, then, we surrender to Him in humble love, He will spread His messianic power over us. We will bear Him within ourselves and sing a triumphal hymn, as did the Righteous Elder Simeon. But if we let the long years of our life extinguish from our hearts the hope of so great a salvation, we will end in shipwreck. If eternity ceases to be our indispensable inspiration whereby our earthly existence is worthily fulfilled, we will inevitably conform to the gloomy reality of the fallen world that surrounds us. And therein lies the tragedy of humanity.

The Lord has given us a sacred deposit which we hold on trust, and He expects us to present it to Him undefiled in that day, when He shall come again to judge the world with justice and goodness. As we have said, there can be no neutrality of attitude; if we surrender to Him, we too will sing a song of victory like St. Simeon, because there will never be a greater day than that day when we shall meet the Lord, our Maker and our Redeemer. This is the great hope that keeps alive our hearts in spite of the hardships of priesthood. We must remember that we are partakers of the priesthood of Christ, and that His priesthood in this world is one of suffering. Therefore, we must not allow ourselves to become fainthearted in trials and tribulations, but rather stir up our expectation through prayer and worship. The gift which God bestowed on us at our ordination will then continually revive our heart, and firmly establish it in the hope of the good things to come.

This world in which we now live, no matter how beautiful it may be, is like a veil that separates us from both the kingdom of God and the kingdom of darkness. There are times, however, when the shadow of the kingdom of darkness is cast over us; sometimes, we receive the luminous rays of the kingdom of light, which console us and sustain us. We must simply keep the gift of God in our heart, so as to be able to stand in that day when the Lord will shake heaven and earth. Then all those things which are created will pass away, and only those things that are marked by the uncreated grace of His Cross and Resurrection will remain forever.

Just before His Passion, the Lord said, 'Now is the judgment of this world' (John 12:3). As He was hanging upon the Cross, the world was indeed judged. He was silent, but the whole creation lent Him its voice. We know that the sun was darkened, rocks were split, and the graves of the dead were opened; and other prodigious things happened (cf. Matt. 27:45–53). And all those who were present who bore not the light of His grace in their hearts 'smote their breasts, and returned' (Luke 23:48). They could not bear the scene of His crucifixion. The only two people who were able to stand at the foot of the Cross were the Lord's Mother and St. John the Divine. For He Who was dead upon the Cross was alive in their hearts, and He it was Who enabled them to stand unshakeable in that dreadful hour, though they were of course in great pain.

If we, too, love God's first appearing, and if we treasure the gift which has been bestowed upon us, a wondrous light will shine in our hearts, inspiring the hope and expectation of His Second Coming. This light, small as it may be now, will become an opening into the everlasting kingdom of light when the Lord comes again in glory; and then, with all the saints, we shall, like Righteous Simeon, sing a hymn of triumph: 'Blessed is He Who has come and is coming again in the Name of the Lord.' Amen.

NOTES

* Homily given during the Divine Liturgy on the last day of the Clergy Brotherhood Retreat, Friday, February 9, 2007.

1. See Archimandrite Zacharias, *The Enlargement of the Heart: "Be ye also enlarged"* (2 Corinthians 6:13) *in the Theology of Saint Silouan the Athonite and Elder Sophrony of Essex* (South Canaan, PA: Mount Thabor Publishing, 2006), pp. 192–195.